Gastric Bypass Cookbook

The Best of The Gastric Bypass Diet Recipes

BY: Valeria Ray

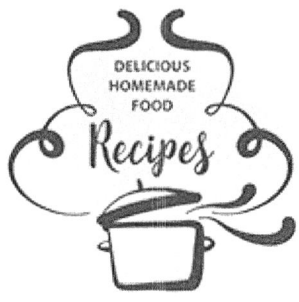

License Notes

Copyright © 2019 Valeria Ray All Rights Reserved

All rights to the content of this book are reserved by the Author without exception unless permission is given stating otherwise.

The Author have no claims as to the authenticity of the content and the Reader bears all responsibility and risk when following the content. The Author is not liable for any reparations, damages, accidents, injuries or other incidents occurring from the Reader following all or part of this publication.

A Special Reward for Purchasing My Book!

Thank you, cherished reader, for purchasing my book and taking the time to read it. As a special reward for your decision, I would like to offer a gift of free and discounted books directly to your inbox. All you need to do is fill in the box below with your email address and name to start getting amazing offers in the comfort of your own home. You will never miss an offer because a reminder will be sent to you. Never miss a deal and get great deals without having to leave the house! Subscribe now and start saving!

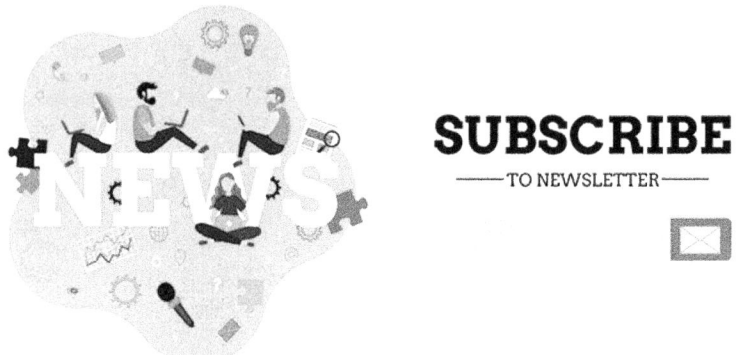

https://valeria-ray.gr8.com

Contents

Homemade Gastric Bypass Diet Recipes 8

Chapter I: Stage One 9

    (1) Butternut Squash Creamy Soup 10

    (2) Banana Blue Smoothie with Green Spinach 13

    (3) Refreshing Gingery Carrot Juice 15

Chapter II: Stage Two 17

    (4) Softened Avocado and Pineapples 18

    (5) Spinach Apple Puree 20

    (6) Milky Roasted Pumpkin 22

Chapter III: Stage Three 24

    (7) Creamy Green Peas 25

    (8) Mashed Potato Garlic 28

    (9) Smooth White Beans with Lemon 31

Chapter IV: Stage Four-Breakfast 33

(10) Soft and Fluffy Pancake 34

(11) Pumpkin Oatmeal Porridge.. 37

(12) Baked Tofu in Cup... 39

(13) Onion and Cheese Egg Muffins 42

(14) Zucchini Muffins with Broccoli 45

(15) Sweet Potato Pancakes 48

(16) Scrambled Tofu Veggie.. 51

(17) Apple Oatmeal with Cinnamon 54

(18) Spinach Mushroom Quiche 56

(19) No Flour Pumpkin Bread.. 59

Chapter V: Stage Four-Lunch 62

(20) Soft Pork Meatloaf... 63

(21) Baked Chicken with Mashed Avocado 66

(22) Avocado Chicken Salads 69

(23) Tomato Beef Roll 72

(24) Salmon Cheese Fritter 75

(25) Chicken Zucchini Noodle 78

(26) Seafood Veggie Soup 81

(27) Spinach Creamy Chicken 84

(28) Simple Tuna Garlic 87

(29) Black Beans Smooth Soup... 90

Chapter VI: Stage Four-Dinner 93

(30) Lentil Loaf Barbecue 94

(31) Sweet Brown Chicken Breast...................................... 97

(32) Sweet Sour Beef Tender with Broccoli 99

(33) Turkey Soup Mushroom... 102

(34) Baked Chicken Balls with Cheese Sauce 104

(35) Sautéed Shrimps Garlic 108

(36) Beans Soup with Enchilada Sauce............................ 110

(37) Tomato Beef Casserole 113

(38) Savory Steamed Fish.. 116

(39) Mixed Vegetables Tender... 119

Chapter VII: Stage Four-Snack and Dessert.......................... 122

    (40) Mango Tropical Salsa 123

    (41) Dense Oatmeal Cake 125

    (42) Roasted Chickpeas.. 128

    (43) Vanilla Melon Pudding 130

    (44) Silky Cheese with Cinnamon 132

    (45) Roasted Cauliflower Garlic 135

    (46) Orange Mango Popsicles... 137

    (47) Strawberry Sorbet with Ricotta Cheese..................... 139

    (48) Meat Cups and Creamy Topping.............................. 141

    (49) Lemon Mug Cake 144

About the Author... 147

Author's Afterthoughts... 149

Homemade Gastric Bypass Diet Recipes

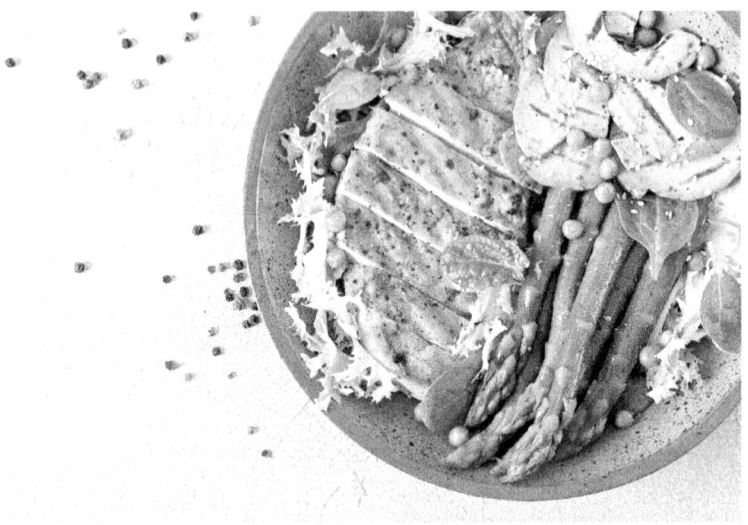

Chapter I: Stage One

MMMMMMMMMMMMMMMMMMMMMMMMMMMMMM

(1) Butternut Squash Creamy Soup

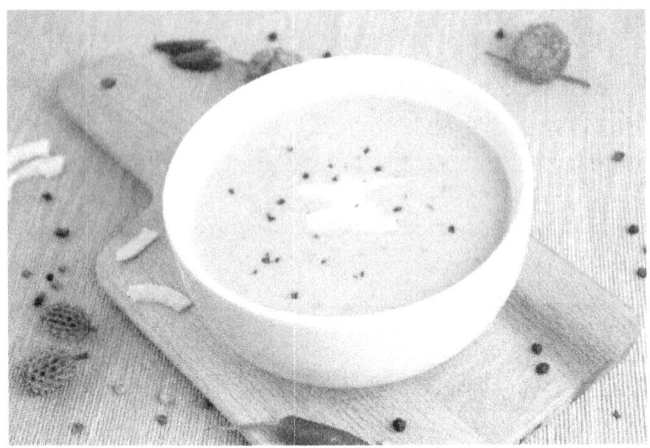

Soft and creamy is the right description for this butternut squash soup. With all the beneficial content of butternut squash, this light soup will be a good start after having a gastric bypass. As a variation, you can add cinnamon or nutmeg to the soup. Besides that, adding celery to this soup will also be a great touch. It will give a better aroma and taste.

Yield: 1

Preparation Time: 1 hour

List of Ingredients:

- ½ cup diced butternut squash
- ¼ cup chopped onion
- 1 fresh pear
- ¼ tsp. thyme
- ½ tsp. olive oil
- 1-½ tbsp. low sodium chicken broth
- 3 tbsp. skim milk

MMMMMMMMMMMMMMMMMMMMMMMMMMMMMMM

Methods:

1. Preheat an oven to 400 °F and line a baking sheet with aluminum foil.
2. Cut the pear into small diced pieces, then place them on the prepared baking sheet. Spread evenly.
3. Sprinkle chopped onion over the diced pear then top with diced butternut squash.
4. Put the baking sheet into the oven and then bake for 45 minutes or until the butternut squash and the pear are tender.
5. Remove from the oven then transfer to a blender.
6. Add thyme and olive oil to the blender then pour skim milk and chicken broth over the ingredients. Blend until smooth and incorporated.
7. Pour the smooth mixture into a small pan then bring to a simmer.
8. Remove the pan from heat and transfer the soup to a serving dish.
9. Serve and enjoy.

(2) Banana Blue Smoothie with Green Spinach

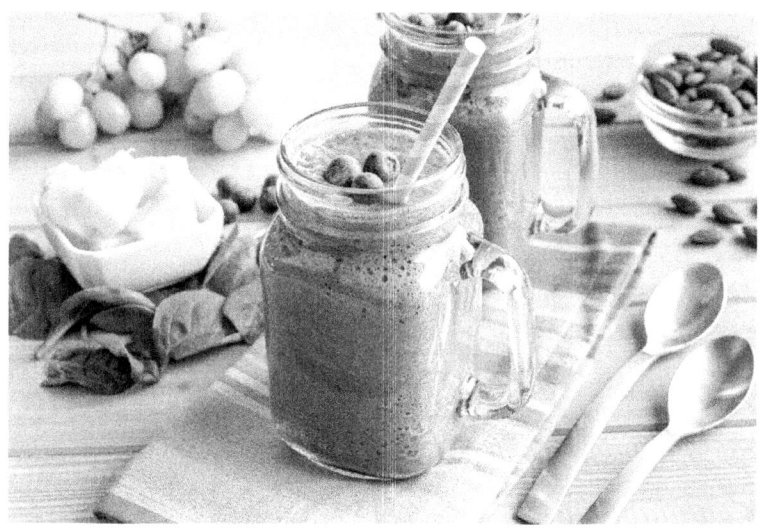

This smoothie is full of protein. With the high nutrient contents of a banana, blueberries, and spinach, this smoothie will be great for you. Another good thing about this smoothie is that you will be surprised to know how blueberry can mask the original taste of spinach. This means that you will have all the benefits of spinach without knowing that it is there!

Yield: 1

Preparation Time: 5 minutes

List of Ingredients:

- 1-cup fresh spinach
- 1 small banana
- ½ cup fresh blueberries
- ½ cup skim milk
- ½ tbsp. protein powder

Methods:

1. Place the spinach in a blender followed by protein powder.
2. Peel the banana, then cut it into slices.
3. Add the sliced banana and fresh blueberries to the blender. Then pour skim milk over the ingredients.
4. Blend the ingredients on high until smooth, then transfer to a serving glass.
5. Serve and enjoy right away.

(3) Refreshing Gingery Carrot Juice

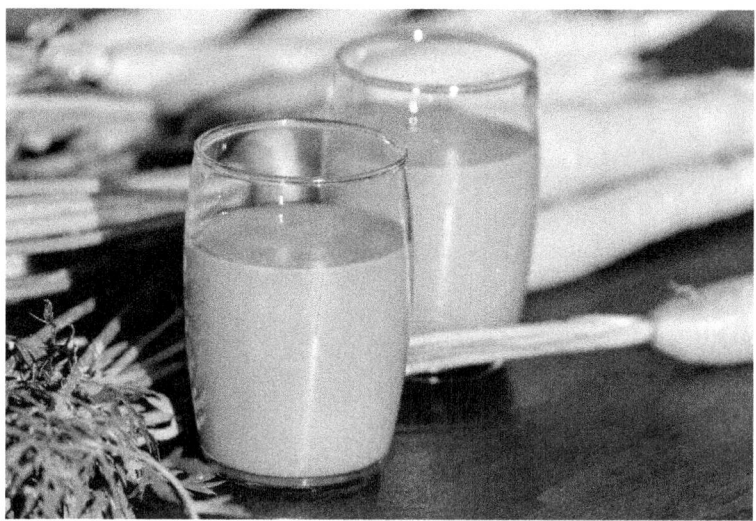

Known as one of the world's healthiest vegetables, carrots are really good to be involved in your after-operation meal plan. With the high content of vitamins and mineral, there is no doubt that carrot can fulfill your need for nutrients. Combining carrot with ginger will not only give you essential health benefits but also a great warm taste.

Size: 1

Preparation Time: 3 Minutes

List of Ingredients:

- 8 medium carrots
- ½ tsp. ginger
- 1 small beet

MMMMMMMMMMMMMMMMMMMMMMMMMMMMMM

Methods:

1. Wash the carrots then place in a bowl. Set aside.
2. Peel the beet then place in the same bowl with the carrots.
3. Prepare your electric juicer then place and press the carrot and beet one at a time.
4. Add ginger to the juice then mix well.
5. Serve and enjoy immediately.

Chapter II: Stage Two

MMMMMMMMMMMMMMMMMMMMMMMMMMMMMMMMM

(4) Softened Avocado and Pineapples

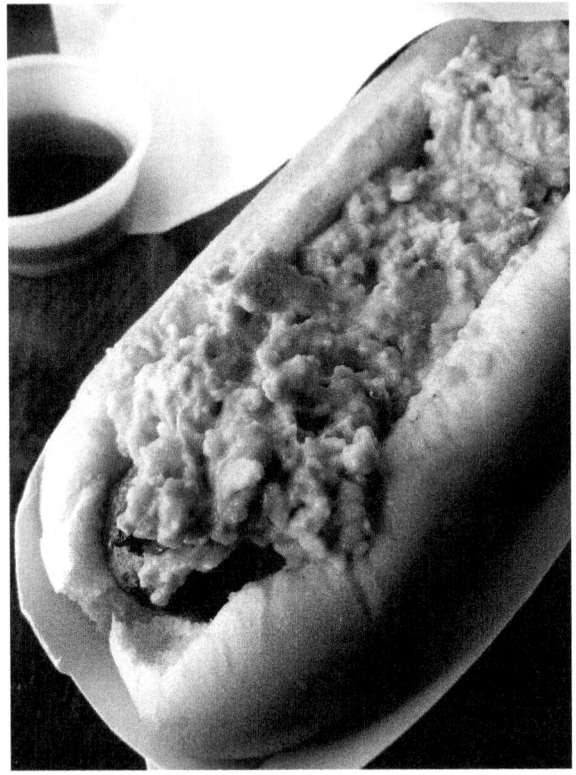

Avocado is a perfect fruit for the second stage after a gastric bypass. This fruit is incredibly smooth and easy to blend with other fruits. This avocado and pineapple puree serves an ideal consistency for your body, which is just learning to adapt to the new changes it's gone through.

Yield: 1

Preparation Time: 10 minutes

List of Ingredients:

- 1 cup pineapple chunks
- 1 ripe avocado
- 3 tbsp. skim milk
- ¾ tbsp. grated non-fat cheese

MMMMMMMMMMMMMMMMMMMMMMMMMMMMMMM

Methods:

1. Cut the avocado into halves, then discard the seed.
2. Scoop out the avocado flesh, then put it in the blender.
3. Add the pineapple chunks. Pour skim milk over everything.
4. Sprinkle grated non-fat cheese over the avocado and pineapple then blend until smooth.
5. Transfer the smooth mixture to a serving bowl then pour the liquid into a serving dish.
6. Enjoy!

(5) Spinach Apple Puree

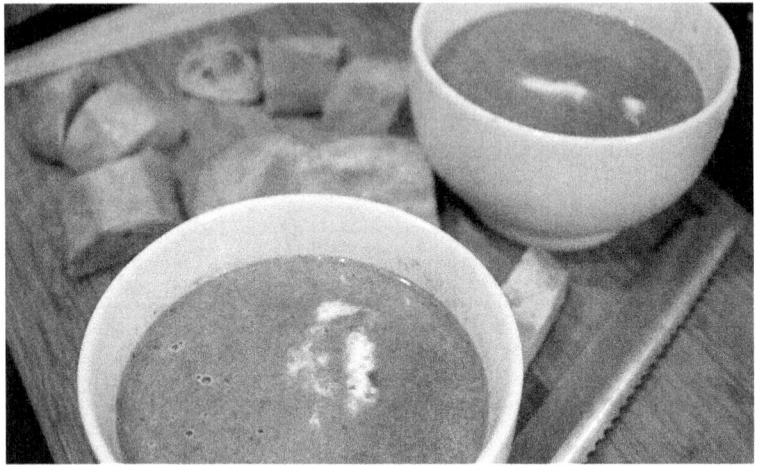

There is no doubt that apple and spinach contain great nutrients for the body. That is why; this spinach and apple puree becomes a perfect choice for the second stage after having a gastric bypass. Cinnamon and ginger in this recipe make this puree tastes amazing!

Yield: 1

Preparation Time: 5 minutes

List of Ingredients:

- 1 fresh apple
- 1 cup chopped spinach
- ½ cup water
- ½ tsp. cinnamon
- ¼ tsp. ginger

MMMMMMMMMMMMMMMMMMMMMMMMMMMMMMM

Methods:

1. Preheat a saucepan over medium heat.
2. Cut the apple into cubes or slices then place in the saucepan.
3. Season with cinnamon and ginger then pour water into the saucepan. Bring to a boil.
4. Reduce the heat and cook for about 3 minutes or until the apple is tender.
5. Add the chopped spinach to the saucepan, then cook until the spinach is just wilted.
6. Remove from the heat then transfer the mixture to a blender. Blend until smooth.
7. Pour the mixture into a bowl, then serve right away.
8. Enjoy.

(6) Milky Roasted Pumpkin

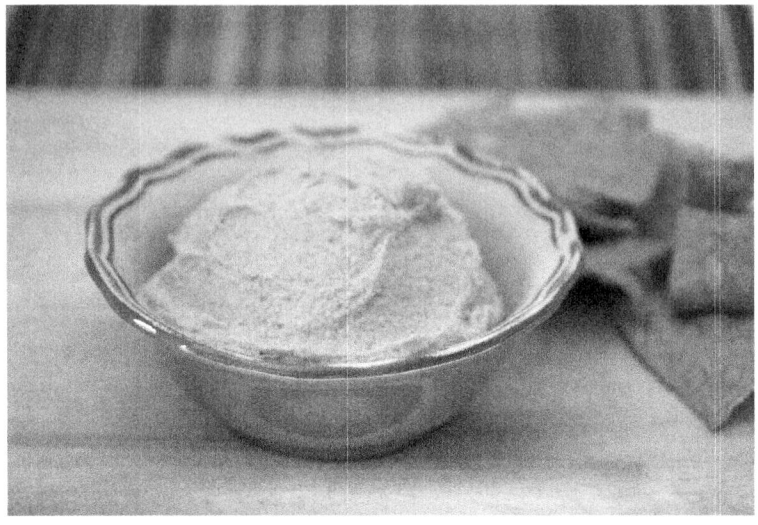

Pumpkin contains lots of good nutrients for the body, this humble vegetable becomes a perfect option to support the recovery process after having a gastric bypass. Besides that, the pumpkin is also delicious. Make sure that you roast the pumpkin until tender before mashing it!

Yield: 1

Preparation Time: 25 minutes

List of Ingredients:

- 1 cup cubed pumpkin
- 1 ½ tsp. coconut oil
- 2 tbsp. skim milk
- 1 tsp. cinnamon
- ¼ tsp. pepper

MMMMMMMMMMMMMMMMMMMMMMMMMMMMMM

Methods:

1. Preheat an oven to 400 °F and line a baking sheet with parchment paper.
2. Spread the pumpkin on the prepared baking sheet then drizzle coconut oil over the pumpkin. Toss to combine.
3. Bake for approximately 25 minutes or until tender.
4. Remove the roasted pumpkin from the oven then transfer to a food processor.
5. Pour skim milk over the pumpkin then season with pepper and cinnamon.
6. Process the pumpkin until smooth and creamy then transfer to a serving dish.
7. Serve and enjoy.

Chapter III: Stage Three

MMMMMMMMMMMMMMMMMMMMMMMMMMMMM

(7) Creamy Green Peas

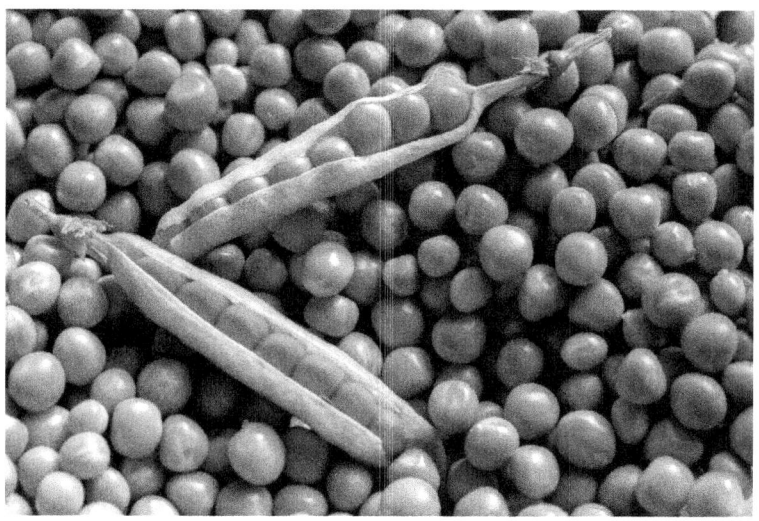

Some say that green pea is the poor's meat as it is cheap. However, this recipe shows that green peas cannot be underestimated. Try this recipe and prove that these creamy green peas really lend a wonderful taste and smooth texture. For an extra refreshing sensation, add fresh mint leaves to this puree.

Yield: 1

Preparation Time: 15 minutes

List of Ingredients:

- ½ cup frozen peas
- 1 tsp. olive oil
- 1 tbsp. chopped onion
- ½ tsp. minced garlic
- A pinch of salt
- ¼ tsp. pepper
- 2 tbsp. non-fat sour cream

MMMMMMMMMMMMMMMMMMMMMMMMMMMMMM

Methods:

1. Place the frozen peas in a pot then pour in enough water to cover them. Bring to boil.
2. Once it has reached a boil, reduce the heat. Cook the peas for approximately 2 minutes or until the peas are tender.
3. Drain the peas then set aside.
4. Preheat a pan over medium heat, then pour olive oil into the pan.
5. Stir in minced garlic and chopped onion. Sauté until wilted and aromatic.
6. Add the peas to the pan. Pour non-fat sour cream over the peas.
7. Season with salt and pepper then stir well.
8. Transfer the peas and the liquid to a food processor. Blend until smooth.
9. Place the creamy peas in a serving bowl then serve.
10. Enjoy right away.

(8) Mashed Potato Garlic

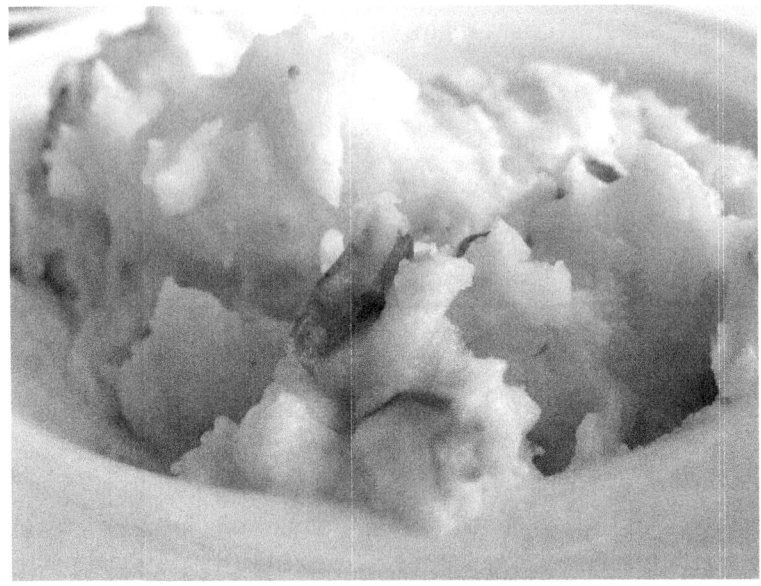

Who doesn't like a mashed potato? This mashed potato is easy but delicious. Use your creativity to enrich this mashed potato. Adding some other herbs to this mashed potato can make it tastier. Rosemary, thyme, nutmeg, and parsley will be suitable choices for this recipe.

Yield: 1

Preparation Time: 30 minutes

List of Ingredients:

- 2 medium potatoes
- 1 tbsp. olive oil
- 2 tbsp. skim milk
- 1 tsp. minced garlic
- ¼ tsp. nutmeg
- ¼ tsp. pepper

MMMMMMMMMMMMMMMMMMMMMMMMMMMMMM

Methods:

1. Peel the potatoes then cut into quarters.
2. Place the potatoes in a steamer. Steam for approximately 20 minutes or until the potatoes are tender.
3. Once the potatoes are tender, take them out of the steamer.
4. Using a potato masher mash the steamed potato until smooth. Set aside.
5. Preheat a saucepan over medium heat then pour olive oil into the saucepan.
6. Stir in minced garlic then sauté until aromatic and lightly golden.
7. Transfer the sautéed garlic together with the olive oil to the mashed potatoes. Pour skim milk over the mashed potato.
8. Season with pepper and nutmeg, then mix well.
9. Serve and enjoy.

(9) Smooth White Beans with Lemon

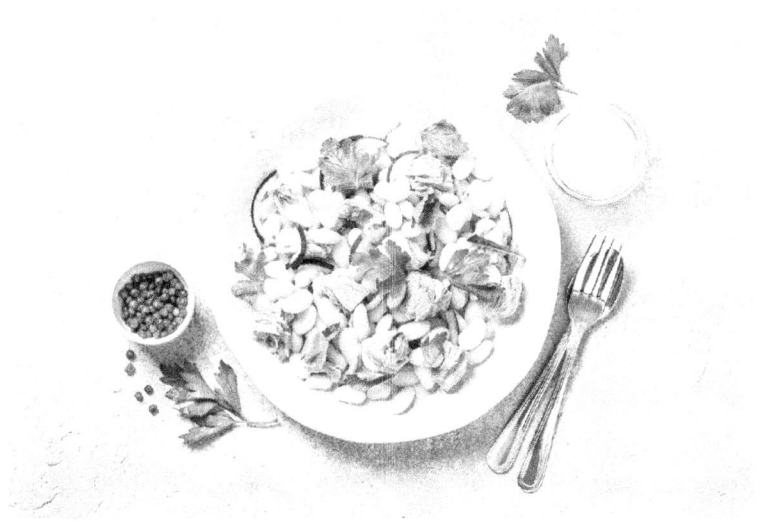

Trust me, this dish is not only very simple and quick but also delicious. The great nutrients in the beans make this dish special, too. All types of beans — such as kidney beans, navy beans, black beans, and pinto beans — fit this recipe. If you have time, cook the beans in advance and chill in an airtight container in the fridge. Take a portion of cooked beans out of the fridge once you want to make this recipe.

Yield: 1

Preparation Time: 10 minutes

List of Ingredients:

- 1 cup cooked white beans
- ½ tsp. minced garlic
- 1 tsp. olive oil
- ¾ tbsp. lemon juice
- ¼ tsp. pepper
- A pinch of salt
- 1 tbsp. diced celeries

Methods:

1. Preheat a skillet over medium heat. Pour olive oil into the skillet.
2. Once it is hot, stir in minced garlic. Sauté until aromatic and lightly golden.
3. Next, add the cooked beans to the skillet, then season with salt and pepper. Mix well.
4. Transfer the seasoned beans to a bowl. Using a potato masher, mash the beans until smooth.
5. Drizzle lemon juice over the mashed beans then add diced celery to the mashed beans. Mix until combined.
6. Serve and enjoy.

Chapter IV: Stage Four-Breakfast

MMMMMMMMMMMMMMMMMMMMMMMMMMMMMM

(10) Soft and Fluffy Pancake

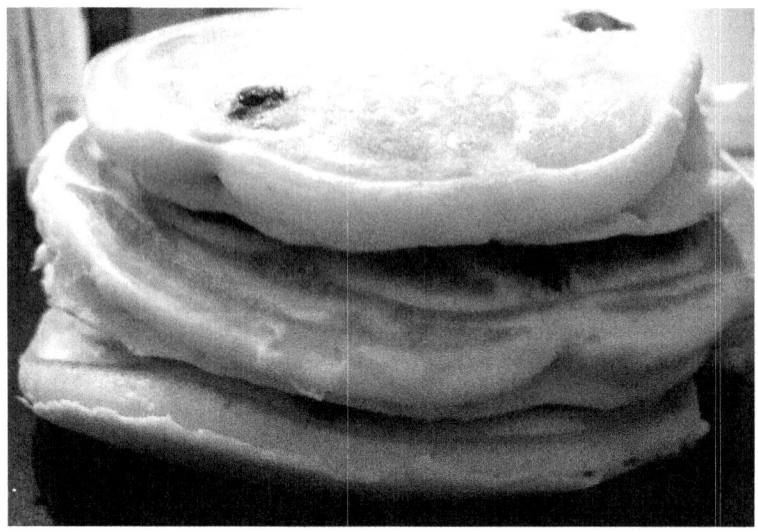

Soft and fluffy are the plus points for this pancake. However, the good things about this pancake do not stop there. For it is made from whole-wheat flour, this pancake serves a high fiber content, which is necessary to prevent constipation. Complete the delicacy of this pancake with some additional toppings as you desire.

Yield: 4

Preparation Time: 15 minutes

List of Ingredients:

- ½ cup organic egg white
- ½ tsp. cinnamon
- 2 tsp. vanilla
- ½ cup whole-wheat flour
- ½ cup water
- ¾ tsp. baking soda

MMMMMMMMMMMMMMMMMMMMMMMMMMMMMM

Methods:

1. Place whole-wheat flour in a bowl, then add cinnamon, baking soda, and vanilla.
2. Pour water into the dry mixture. Stir until incorporated and smooth. Set aside.
3. Pour the egg whites into a mixing bowl then use an electric mixer mix to create soft peaks.
4. Stir the egg whites into the whole-wheat mixture, then mix until smooth and fluffy.
5. Preheat a saucepan over medium heat then coat with cooking spray.
6. Pour 2 tbsp. of the batter then make a thin pancake. Repeat with the remaining batter.
7. Arrange the pancakes on a serving dish then serve.
8. Enjoy!

(11) Pumpkin Oatmeal Porridge

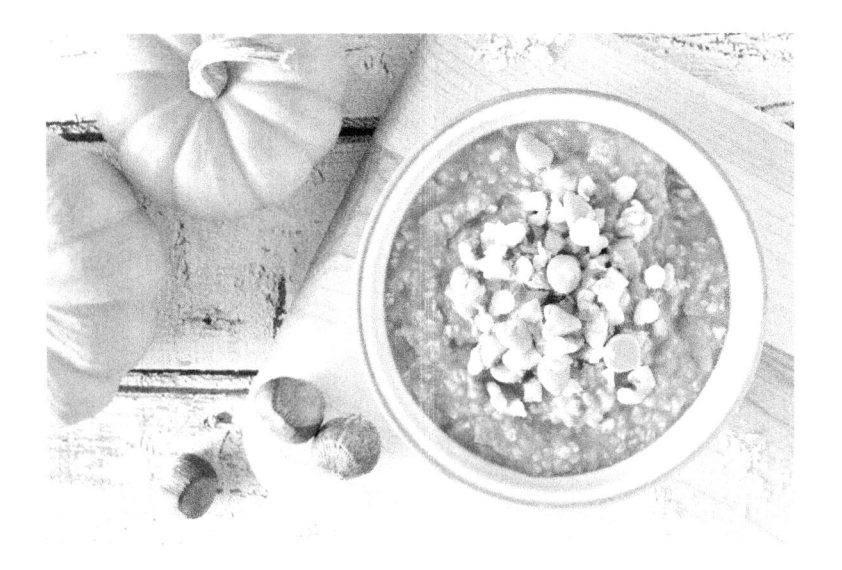

Known as a great antioxidant with fantastic health benefits, pumpkin is a perfect choice for your recovery process after having a gastric bypass. With oatmeal as a partner, this dish will be a very great source of fiber and protein. Serve this dish as a start to your day and enjoy warm!

Yield: 1

Preparation Time: 15 minutes

List of Ingredients:

- 4 tbsp. non-fat milk
- ¾ cup water
- 4 tbsp. old-fashioned oats
- ¼ tsp. cinnamon
- ¼ tsp. nutmeg
- 3 tbsp. pumpkin puree
- ½ scoop vanilla protein powder

Methods:

1. Pour ½ cup water and milk into a saucepan, then bring to boil.
2. Once it is boiling, stir in oatmeal then season with cinnamon and nutmeg. Bring to a simmer.
3. After that, add the pumpkin puree to the saucepan. Stir to combine.
4. In another bowl, combine the vanilla protein powder with the remaining water. Stir until incorporated. Use a blender if it is necessary.
5. Pour the protein mixture over the pumpkin oatmeal then stir well.
6. Serve and enjoy.

(12) Baked Tofu in Cup

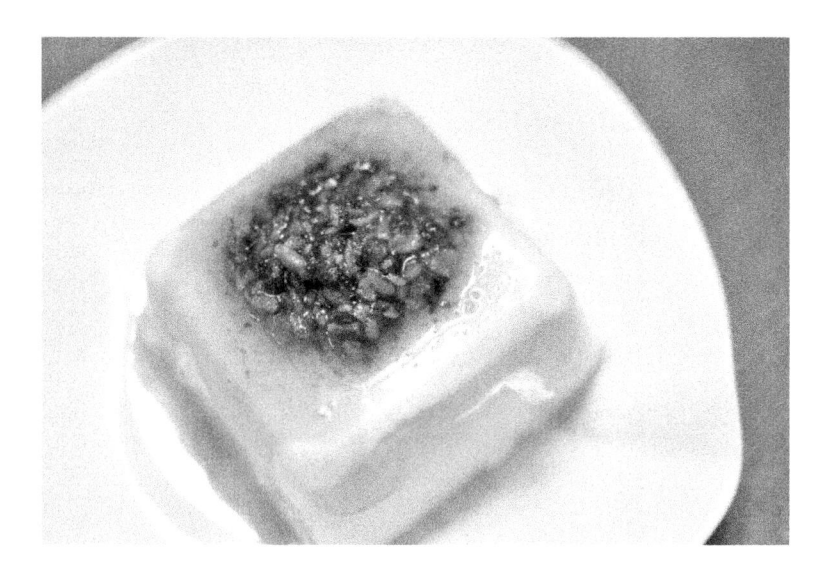

This dish is magical. It serves crispy and crunchy texture outside but soft and smooth inside. Eating this baked tofu with vegetables in the morning will give you enough energy for your busy day. Not only for breakfast, but this baked tofu is also great to be consumed as a snack.

Yield: 4

Preparation Time: 30 minutes

List of Ingredients:

- 1 lb. tofu
- ½ cup diced tomatoes
- 1 cup chopped kale
- ½ cup ground chicken
- 2 organic eggs
- 2 tsp. minced garlic
- ½ tsp. pepper

MMMMMMMMMMMMMMMMMMMMMMMMMMMMMM

Methods:

1. Preheat an oven to 350 °F and prepare 8 muffin cups. Coat with cooking spray then set aside.
2. Place the tofu in a food processor, then add eggs and ground chicken to the food processor.
3. Season with pepper and minced garlic. Blend until smooth.
4. Transfer the tofu mixture to a bowl, then stir diced tomatoes and chopped kale into the bowl. Mix until just combined.
5. Fill each muffin cup with the tofu mixture, then bake for approximately 25 minutes.
6. Once the tofu is set and lightly golden, remove from the oven and let them cool.
7. Take the tofu from the cups and arrange on a serving dish.
8. Serve and enjoy!

(13) Onion and Cheese Egg Muffins

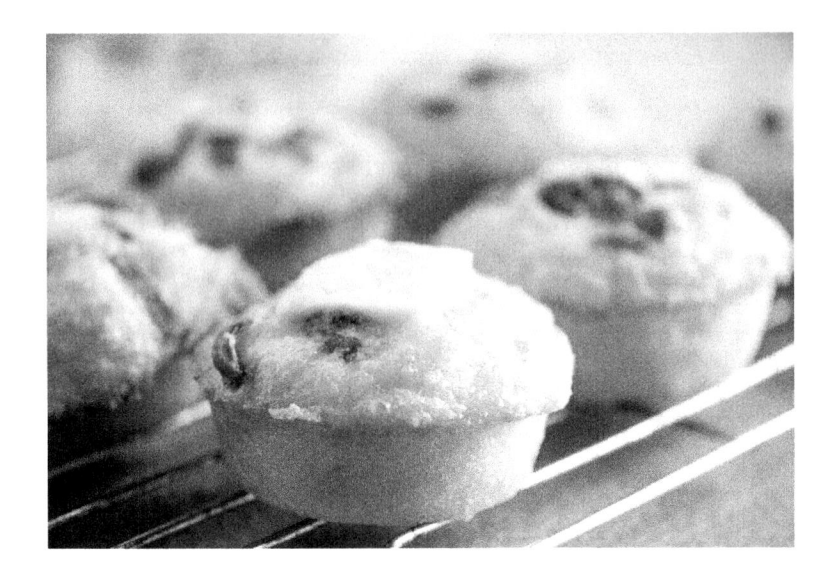

These egg muffins are perfect for a busy morning. The ingredients needed in this recipe are very easy to grab and usually available in your refrigerator. The egg already contains protein which is great to consume after a gastric bypass. However, to enhance the nutrient content, you can add any kind of vegetable or lean ground meat as you desire.

Yield: 4

Preparation Time: 25 minutes

List of Ingredients:

- 8 organic eggs
- 3 tbsp. coconut flour
- ½ tsp. olive oil
- ¼ cup chopped onion
- ¼ cup grated skim Mozzarella cheese

MMMMMMMMMMMMMMMMMMMMMMMMMMMMMMM

Methods:

1. Preheat an oven to 400 °F and coat 4 muffin tins with cooking oil.
2. Crack the eggs into your bowl.
3. Add the coconut flour to the eggs, then whisk until the flour is completely dissolved. Set aside.
4. Preheat a skillet over medium heat, then pour olive oil into it.
5. Once it is hot, stir in the chopped onion and sauté until aromatic. Remove from heat.
6. Add the onion to the egg mixture then stir well.
7. Divide the egg mixture into the prepared muffin cups then sprinkle grated skim Mozzarella cheese on top.
8. Bake the egg muffins for approximately 20 minutes or until the egg is set.
9. Once it is done, take the egg muffins out from the oven then let them cool for a few minutes.
10. Arrange the egg muffins on a serving dish then enjoy!

(14) Zucchini Muffins with Broccoli

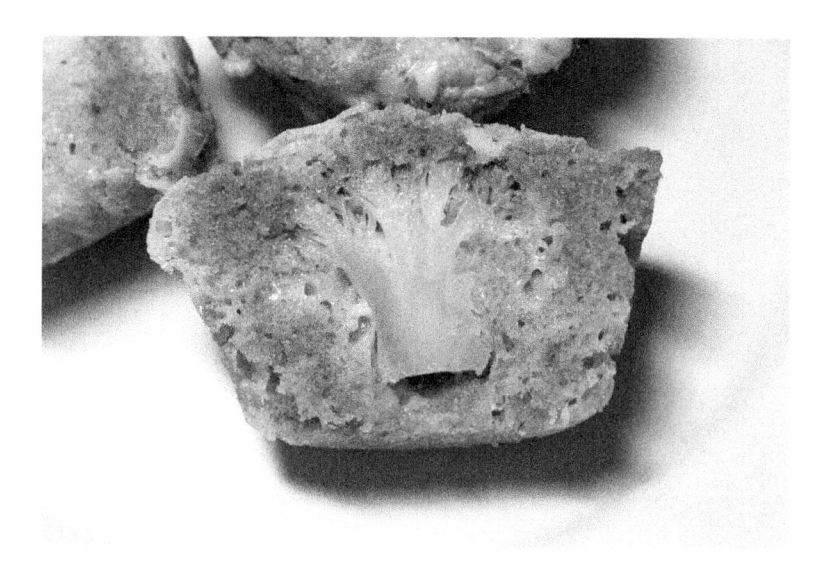

This is a muffin that you can consume with no guilty feeling. With no sugar, no oil, and no flour, there is no doubt that this muffin is ideal for the weight loss. Zucchini — which is rich in great nutrients for the body — has countless benefits for the body. Make sure to buy the fresh zucchinis with a firm texture and bright color.

Yield: 4

Preparation Time: 60 minutes

List of Ingredients:

- 1¼ cups grated zucchini
- 8 broccoli florets
- 1¼ cups oats
- 1 medium ripe banana
- 2 organic eggs
- ¼ cup applesauce
- 1 tsp. baking powder
- 1 tsp. cinnamon

MMMMMMMMMMMMMMMMMMMMMMMMMMMMMM

Methods:

1. Preheat an oven to 350 °F and prepare 8 muffin cups. Coat with cooking spray then set aside.
2. Place the oats in a food processor then process until they become a flour-like consistency. Set aside.
3. Peel the banana, then mash until smooth.
4. Crack the eggs, then pour them over the mashed banana.
5. Add applesauce, grated zucchini, and cinnamon. Mix until incorporated.
6. Combine the oat flour with baking powder. Mix with the liquid mixture.
7. Fill each muffin cup with the batter, then put a broccoli floret in each muffin.
8. Bake the muffins for approximately 40 minutes or until the top of the muffins are lightly golden.
9. Insert a skewer into the muffins and when it comes out clean, it means that the muffins are completely cooked.
10. Remove the muffins from the oven, then let them cool for a few minutes.
11. Arrange on a serving dish then enjoy.

(15) Sweet Potato Pancakes

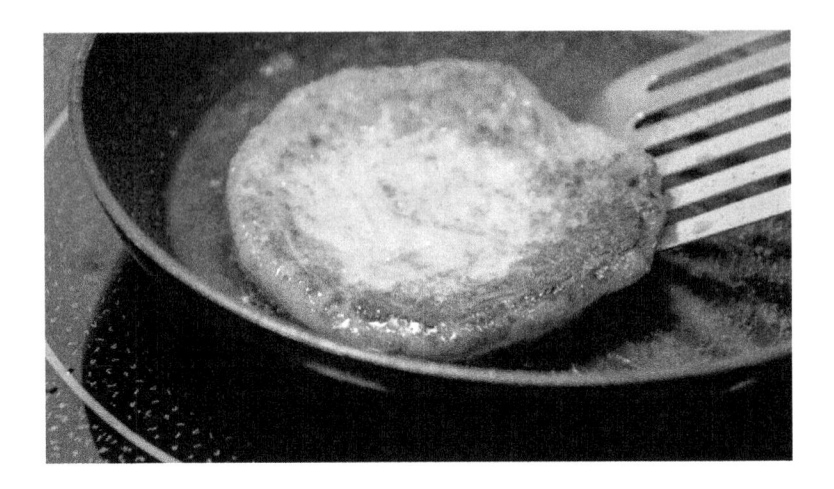

It is the time to let the sweet potato take a role in your healthy breakfast. As a source of fiber and healthy carbs, sweet potato is a good partner for your weight-loss goals. This pancake is another great way to consume the sweet potato. You will be amazed by the smooth and soft texture of this pancake. Have this sweet potato pancake with non-fat whipped cream or fresh fruit.

Yield: 4

Preparation Time: 25 minutes

List of Ingredients:

- 1 lb. sweet potatoes
- 2 organic eggs
- 3 tbsp. whole-wheat flour
- ½ tsp. pepper
- 1 tsp. garlic powder
- 3 tbsp. canola oil

MMMMMMMMMMMMMMMMMMMMMMMMMMMMMMM

Methods:

- Preheat a steamer over medium heat, then place peeled sweet potatoes in it. Steam until tender.
- Once the sweet potatoes are tender, remove from the steamer. Using a potato masher, mash until smooth.
- Place the mashed sweet potatoes in a bowl then add eggs and flour to the bowl.
- Season with pepper and garlic powder, then mix well.
- Shape the sweet potato mixture into thin patties then set aside.
- Preheat a saucepan over medium heat then pour canola oil into it.
- Place the shaped sweet potato in the saucepan then cook until lightly golden.
- Flip the sweet potato pancakes then cook again until both sides of the sweet potato pancakes are lightly golden. Repeat with the rest of the batter.
- Once they are done, arrange the sweet potato pancakes on a serving dish, then serve.
- Enjoy!

(16) Scrambled Tofu Veggie

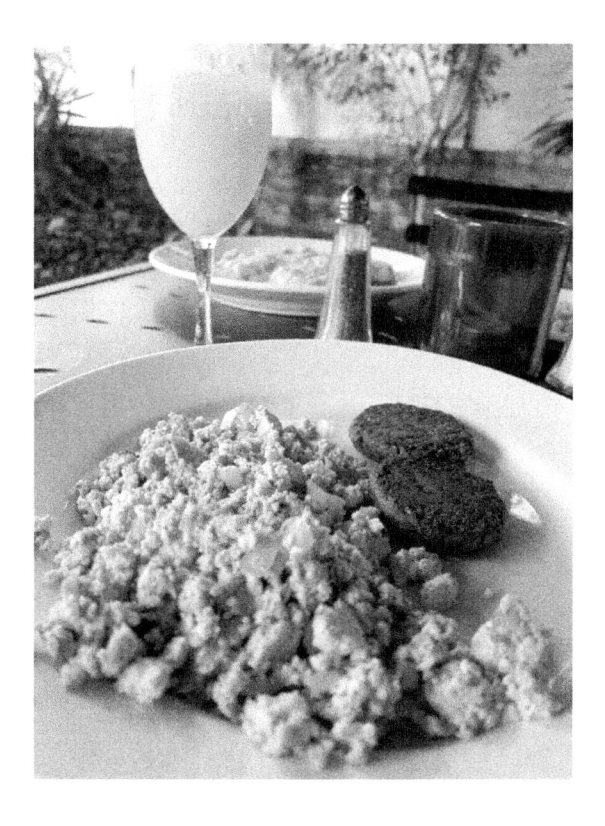

There are a lot of kinds of healthy breakfasts. However, if you want something savory, we suggest that you give this scrambled tofu recipe a try. Served with vegetables, this scrambled tofu not only offers great taste and quick cooking time but also plenty of health benefits. Being low in fats but high in protein, tofu is a perfect support for your weight loss program.

Yield: 4

Preparation Time: 10 minutes

List of Ingredients:

- 3 cups diced tofu
- 2 organic eggs
- 1 cup chopped kale
- ½ cup diced tomatoes
- 2 tsp. olive oil
- 1½ tsp. garlic powder
- ½ tsp. pepper

MMMMMMMMMMMMMMMMMMMMMMMMMMMMMM

Methods:

1. Crack the eggs into a bowl. Mix until incorporated.
2. Preheat a skillet over medium heat then pour olive oil into it.
3. Pour the beaten eggs into the skillet then add the diced tofu to it. Quickly stir the egg and tofu until scramble forms.
4. Add chopped kale and diced tomatoes, then season with garlic powder and pepper. Mix until the vegetables are wilted.
5. Remove the scrambled tofu from the heat. Transfer to a serving dish.
6. Serve and enjoy warm.

(17) Apple Oatmeal with Cinnamon

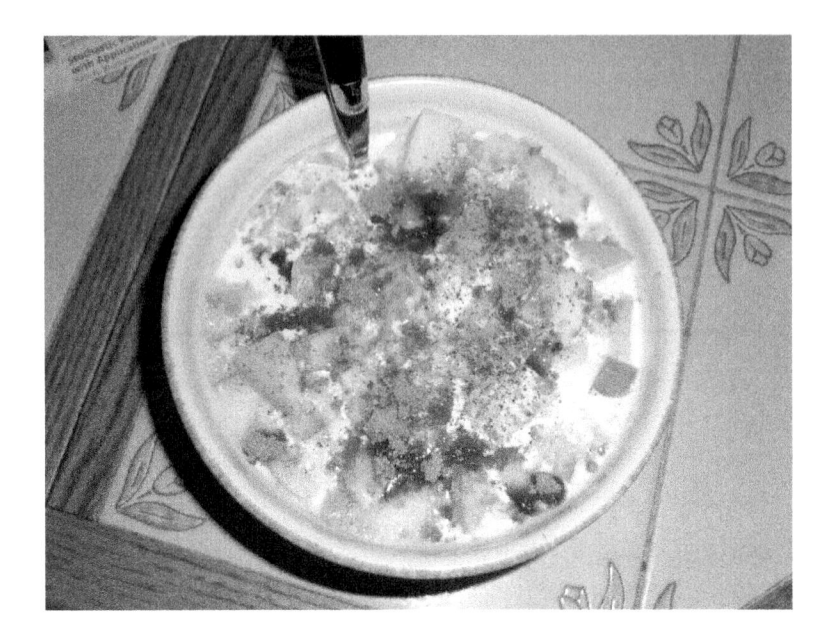

It cannot be denied that this classic breakfast is very healthy. Both apple and oatmeal have a high nutrient content that is important for the body. Besides that, apple gives natural sweetness. That is why additional sugar is not necessary here. For a lighter taste, substitute the skim milk with unsweetened apple juice.

Yield: 1

Preparation Time: 5 minutes

List of Ingredients:

- 1 fresh green apple
- 1 tsp. lemon juice
- ¾ cup skim milk
- ½ cup oats
- ½ tsp. cinnamon

MMMMMMMMMMMMMMMMMMMMMMMMMMMMMMM

Methods:

1. Cut the apple into cubes, then place in a bowl.
2. Drizzle the lemon juice over the cubed apple, then set aside.
3. Pour skim milk into a saucepan and bring it to boil.
4. Once it is boiled, add the oats and apple then bring the mixture to a simmer.
5. Transfer everything to a serving bowl then sprinkle cinnamon on top.
6. Serve and enjoy!

(18) Spinach Mushroom Quiche

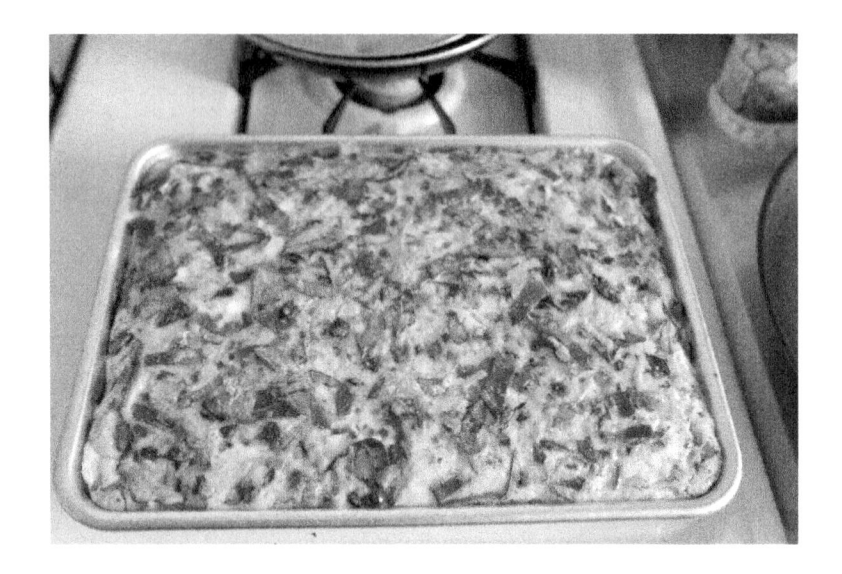

This savory breakfast must be a favorite. Made from organic eggs with additional spinach, mushroom, and cheese, this quiche tastes perfect. As a variation, you can involve other vegetables such as carrots, kale, or broccoli as you desire. To give it an extra cheesy taste, we suggest not grating the Parmesan cheese but cutting the cheese into small cubes. Besides that, you can also sprinkle non-fat grated Mozzarella on top.

Yield: 4

Preparation Time: 50 minutes

List of Ingredients:

- 6 organic eggs
- ½ cup skim milk
- ¼ cup grated Parmesan cheese
- 3 cups chopped spinach
- ½ cup chopped mushroom
- 2 tsp. garlic powder
- ½ tsp. pepper

MMMMMMMMMMMMMMMMMMMMMMMMMMMMMMMMM

Methods:

1. Preheat an oven to 400 °F and coat a disposable aluminum pan with cooking spray.
2. Place the chopped spinach and mushroom in the bottom of the disposable aluminum pan then spread evenly. Set aside.
3. Crack the eggs then place them in a bowl.
4. Pour skim milk in the bowl, then season with garlic powder. Mix well.
5. Pour the egg mixture over the spinach and mushroom then sprinkle grated Mozzarella cheese on top.
6. Bake the spinach and mushroom quiche for about 40 minutes or until the egg mixture is set.
7. When the quiche is done, take it out of the oven.
8. Let the quiche cool for a few minutes then cut into wedges.
9. Serve and enjoy.

(19) No Flour Pumpkin Bread

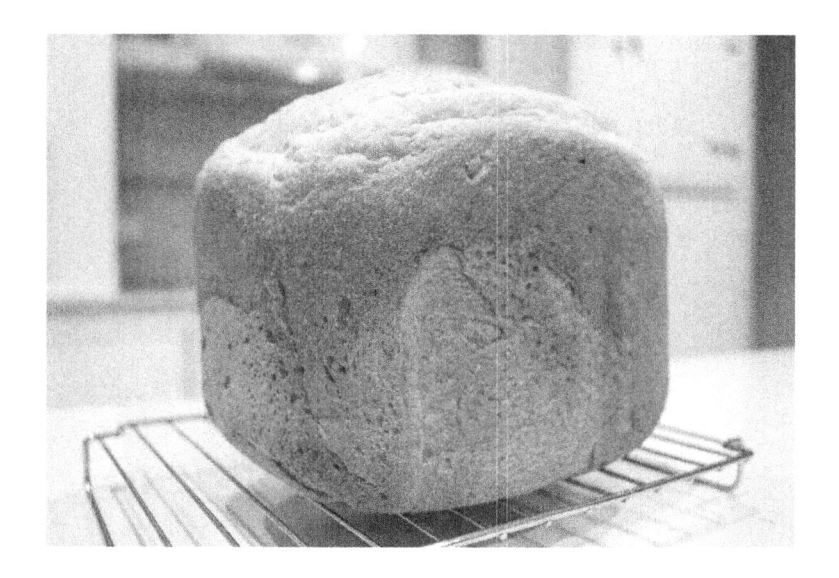

Pumpkin is a sweet but healthy ingredient. It brings delicious taste and delicate texture to every dish it's added to. There is no reason not to include pumpkin in your favorite recipe. This low-carb bread is perfect for your new gut as it is moist, soft, and nutritious. Besides being good for breakfast, this bread is also perfect for your snack time.

Yield: 4

Preparation Time: 35 minutes

List of Ingredients:

- 1 cup quick cooking oats
- 1 cup pumpkin puree
- 3 tbsp. applesauce
- 1 organic egg
- ½ tsp. baking soda
- ¾ tsp. cinnamon

MMMMMMMMMMMMMMMMMMMMMMMMMMMMM

Methods:

1. Preheat an oven to 350 °F and line a loaf pan with parchment paper. Set aside.
2. Place the pumpkin puree and oats in a blender, then add egg, baking soda, applesauce, and cinnamon to the bowl. Using an electric mixer, mix the ingredients until smooth and combined.
3. Transfer the batter to the prepared loaf pan then spread evenly.
4. Bake the pumpkin bread for approximately 30 minutes or until the top of the bread is lightly golden.
5. Insert a toothpick into the bread and if it comes out clean, it means that the bread is completely done.
6. Remove the bread from the oven and let it cool for a few minutes.
7. Take the pumpkin bread out of the loaf pan and cut into slices.
8. Arrange the sliced bread on a serving dish, then serve.
9. Enjoy!

Chapter V: Stage Four-Lunch

MMMMMMMMMMMMMMMMMMMMMMMMMMMMM

(20) Soft Pork Meatloaf

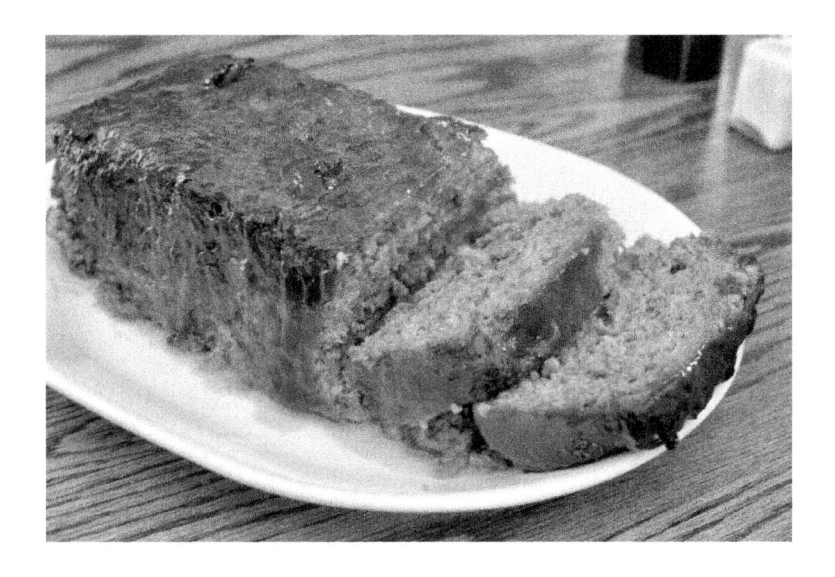

This meatloaf is easy and tasty. It is another way to use ground meat. Not only pork, but beef and poultry also work well with this recipe. To add to the nutrient content, we suggest including vegetables in this meatloaf. However, to keep the meatloaf smooth, it is better to grate the vegetables or cut them into very small pieces.

Yield: 4

Preparation Time: 60 minutes

List of Ingredients:

- 1¼ lbs. lean ground pork
- ¼ cup chopped onion
- ¼ cup tomato puree
- 1 tsp. white vinegar
- 1 organic egg
- 3 tsp. Worcestershire sauce
- ¼ tsp. basil
- 3 tsp. olive oil
- ½ tsp. pepper

MMMMMMMMMMMMMMMMMMMMMMMMMMMMMMM

Methods:

1. Preheat an oven to 350 °F and prepare a baking sheet. Set aside.
2. Place the ground pork, chopped onion, tomato puree, white vinegar, egg, Worcestershire sauce, basil, olive oil, and pepper in a food processor. Process until smooth.
3. Transfer the smooth mixture to a sheet of aluminum foil then shape into a log.
4. Place the meatloaf on the prepared baking sheet then bake for approximately 40 minutes.
5. Once it is done, remove the meatloaf from the oven then let it cool for approximately 10 minutes.
6. Unwrap the meatloaf then cut into thick slices.
7. Arrange on a serving dish, then serve.
8. Enjoy right away.

(21) Baked Chicken with Mashed Avocado

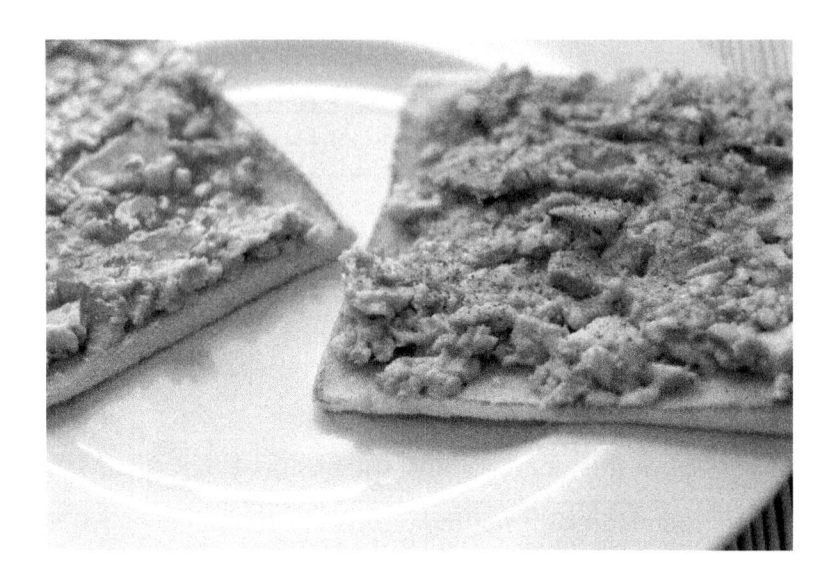

The combination of chicken and avocado is really a perfect idea. Both of them contain a large amount of protein, which is very essential for those who have had a gastric bypass surgery. You can cook the chicken several hours ahead of time. Make sure to mash the avocado just a few minutes before serving.

Yield: 4

Preparation Time: 30 minutes

List of Ingredients:

- 2 lbs. boneless chicken breast
- ½ tsp. salt
- ½ tsp. pepper
- ½ tsp. nutmeg
- 2 tsp. garlic powder
- 2 tbsp. olive oil
- 2 ripe avocados
- 1 tbsp. lemon juice
- 1 ½ tsp. cilantro
- 1½ tsp. avocado oil
- 2 tbsp. chopped onion

MMMMMMMMMMMMMMMMMMMMMMMMMMMMMMM

Methods:

1. Cut the boneless chicken breast into thick slices. Rub the chicken with salt, pepper, nutmeg, and garlic powder. Let the chicken sit for a few minutes.
2. Meanwhile, cut the avocados into halves, then discard the seeds.

3. Scoop out the avocado flesh and put it in a food processor.
4. Add lemon juice, cilantro, chopped onion, and avocado oil to the food processor then process until smooth.
5. Transfer to a container with a lid then chill in the fridge.
6. Preheat a saucepan over medium heat then pour olive oil into it.
7. Once it is hot, put the seasoned chicken on it and cook until it is no longer pink.
8. Flip the chicken and cook until both sides of the chicken are lightly golden brown.
9. Check the doneness of the chicken by pricking the chicken with a knife or fork.
10. Once it is done, take the cooked chicken out from the saucepan then arrange on a serving dish.
11. Top each cooked chicken breast with the avocado mixture then serve.
12. Enjoy!

(22) Avocado Chicken Salads

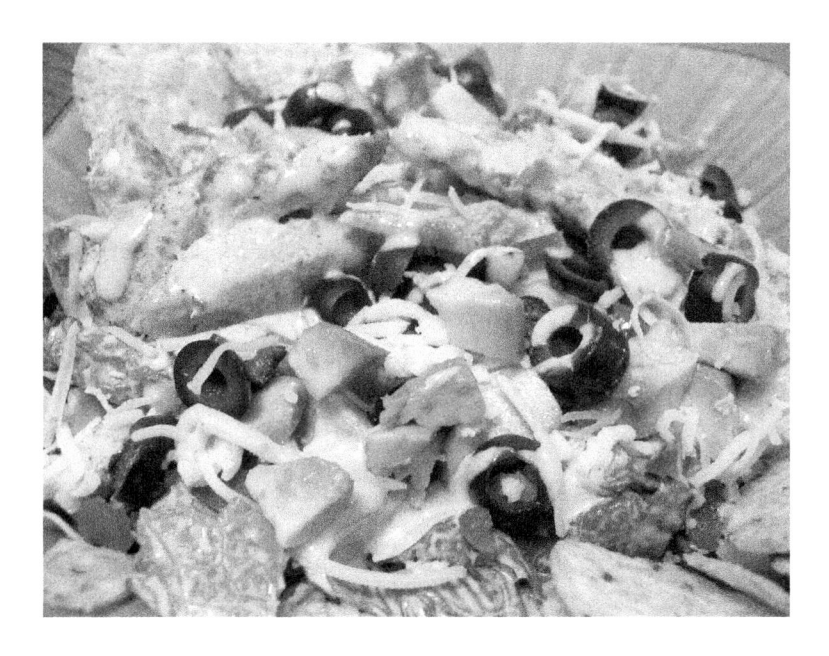

If you like chicken and enjoy avocados, this is the right time to mix these two wonderful ingredients. This salad serves the smooth and creamy chicken combined with the good quality of avocados, for sure, this salad offers you an extra delicacy. Make sure to use the ripe avocados for they are naturally sweet with a smooth texture. Besides that, shrimp give a special touch to this salad. Enjoy!

Yield: 4

Preparation Time: 30 minutes

List of Ingredients:

- 2 ripe avocados
- 1 cup lean ground chicken
- ¼ cup fresh shrimp
- ¼ cup non-fat yogurt
- 1 tsp. minced garlic
- ¼ tsp. pepper
- ¼ cup grated Mozzarella cheese
- ¼ cup diced tomatoes

MMMMMMMMMMMMMMMMMMMMMMMMMMMMMM

Methods:

1. Preheat an oven to 350 °F and prepare a baking sheet. Set aside.
2. Peel the fresh shrimp then discard the head.
3. Place the peeled shrimp in a food processor together with lean ground chicken, minced yogurt, Mozzarella cheese, minced garlic, and pepper. Process until smooth.
4. Cut the avocados into halves then discard the seeds.
5. Fill each halved avocado with the chicken mixture then arrange on the prepared baking sheet.
6. Bake the avocados for approximately 10 minutes then remove from the oven.
7. Arrange the avocados on a serving dish then sprinkle diced tomatoes on top.
8. Serve and enjoy.

(23) Tomato Beef Roll

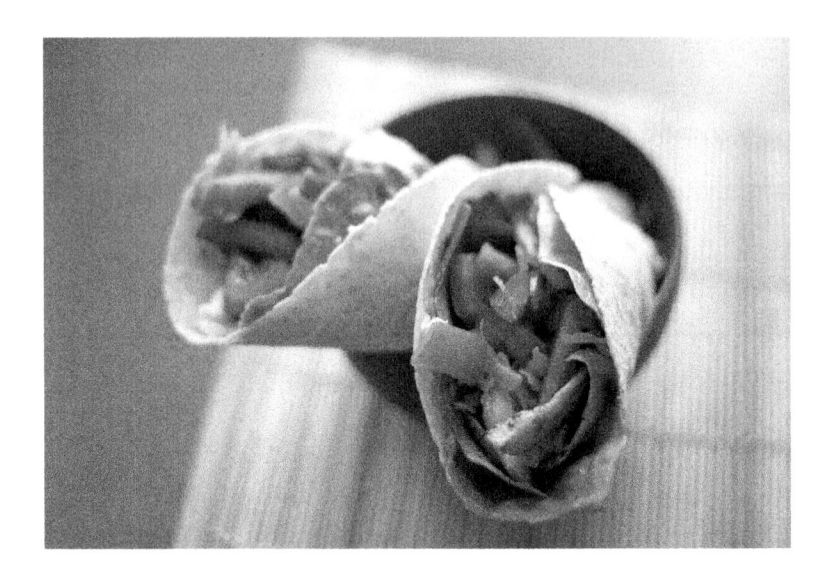

This roll uses beef as the filling since beef is rich in natural protein. You have to choose lean beef for the lower fats content. Combining the beef with tomatoes — that are rich in antioxidant — results in a superfood that is good for the new gastric. Add more herbs to enhance the taste and aroma. Nutmeg, black pepper, turmeric, kaffir lime leaves, or cumin would be an excellent partner for the beef.

Yield: 1

Preparation Time: 20 minutes

List of Ingredients:

- 2 tbsp. ground lean beef
- ½ tsp. olive oil
- 1 tbsp. diced onion
- 1 tbsp. diced tomato
- ½ cup water
- A pinch of salt
- ¼ cup organic egg whites
- 2 tbsp. water
- 1 tbsp. coconut flour

MMMMMMMMMMMMMMMMMMMMMMMMMMMMMM

Methods:

1. Preheat a skillet over medium heat, then brown the lean ground beef.
2. Pour olive oil into the skillet then stir in chopped onion. Sauté together with the browned beef.
3. Pour water over the beef then cook until the water is completely absorbed into the beef.
4. Stir in the diced tomato and season with salt. Remove from heat then set aside.
5. Combine egg whites with water and coconut flour then mix until incorporated.
6. Preheat a pan then coat with cooking spray.
7. Pour a half of the egg mixture over the pan then make an omelet. Repeat with the remaining egg mixture.
8. Place the omelets on a flat surface then drop the beef on top.
9. Roll or fold the omelets then serve.
10. Enjoy!

(24) Salmon Cheese Fritter

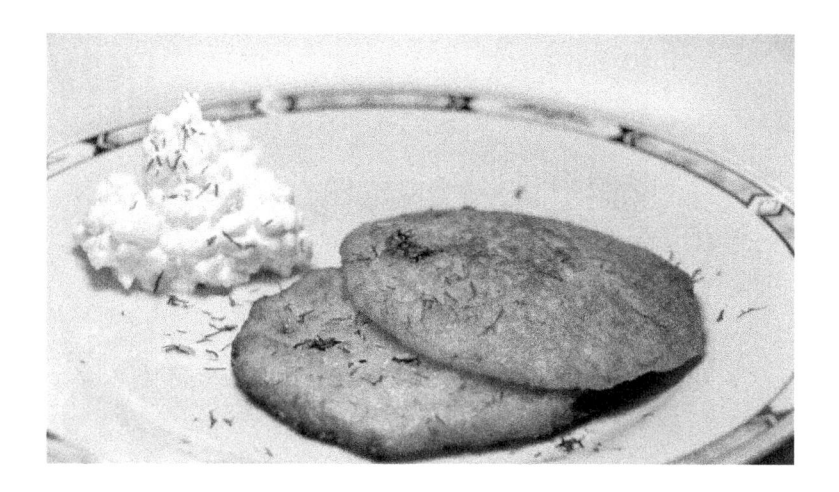

Known as one of the healthiest food in the world, salmon is perfect for those who have just had a gastric bypass. This fritter uses salmon as the main ingredient. With an additional role from cheese and eggs, this fritter doesn't only delicious but also nourishing.

Yield: 4

Preparation Time: 30 minutes

List of Ingredients:

- 2 lbs. salmon fillet
- 2 tbsp. flax meal
- 2 organic eggs
- 2 tbsp. grated Mozzarella cheese
- 1 tsp. onion powder
- 1 tsp. garlic powder

MMMMMMMMMMMMMMMMMMMMMMMMMMMMMM

Methods:

1. Place salmon fillet in a food processor then process until smooth.
2. Add the flax meal, grated Mozzarella cheese, and eggs. Season with the onion powder and garlic powder. Mix well.
3. Preheat an oven to 350 °F and line a baking sheet with parchment paper.
4. Shape the mixture into patty forms then arrange on the prepared baking sheet.
5. Bake the salmon for approximately 10 minutes then flip the salmon fritters.
6. Bake the salmon fritter again for another 10 minutes or until both sides of the salmon fritters are lightly golden.
7. Once it is done, remove from the oven then transfer to a serving dish.
8. Serve and enjoy warm.

(25) Chicken Zucchini Noodle

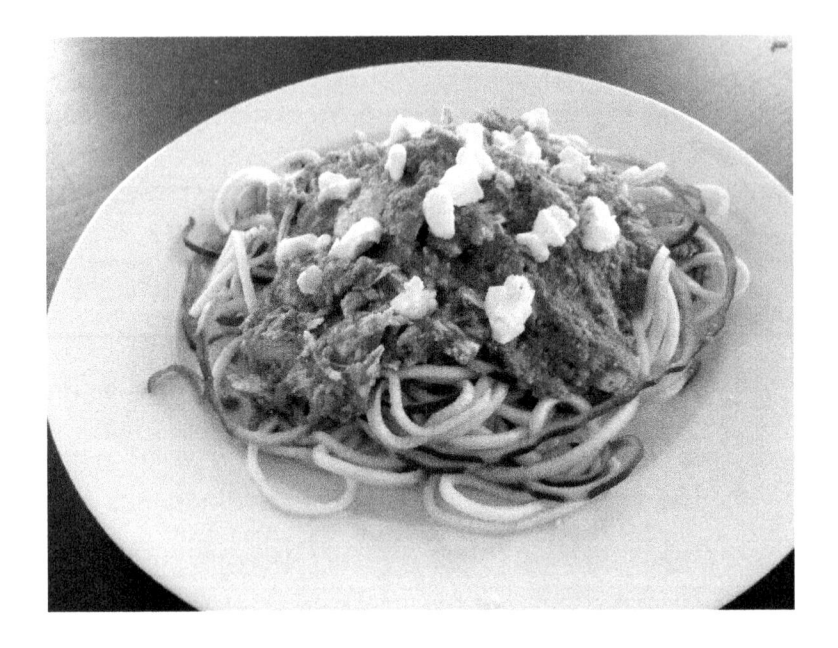

Known as an ingredient that is high in carbs content, the noodle is one of the most avoided ingredients for any kinds of dieting methods. However, this noodle is different. It is made from zucchini, a vegetable that is famous for its healthy nutrient contents. This recipe, for sure, ensures you to have noodles without guilt.

Yield: 4

Preparation Time: 30 minutes

List of Ingredients:

- ¾ lb. boneless chicken breast
- 2 medium zucchinis
- 1 tsp. olive oil
- 2 tsp. minced garlic
- 1 cup chopped green collard
- 1 tbsp. fish sauce
- ¾ tbsp. soy sauce

MMMMMMMMMMMMMMMMMMMMMMMMMMMMMMMM

Methods:

1. Place the boneless chicken breast in a pot, then pour water over the chicken. Bring to a boil.
2. Once it is boiling, reduce the heat then cook until the chicken is tender.
3. Remove from the heat and drain the chicken.
4. Cut the cooked chicken into thin slices, then set aside.
5. Peel the zucchinis. Using a julienne peeler, peel cut the zucchinis into noodle form.
6. Preheat a skillet over medium heat, then pour olive oil into it.
7. Stir in minced garlic then sauté until lightly golden.
8. Add chopped green collard to the skillet then cook until wilted.
9. Stir in the cooked chicken with zucchini noodles then season with fish sauce and soy sauce. Cook until wilted.
10. Transfer to a serving dish then enjoy right away.

(26) Seafood Veggie Soup

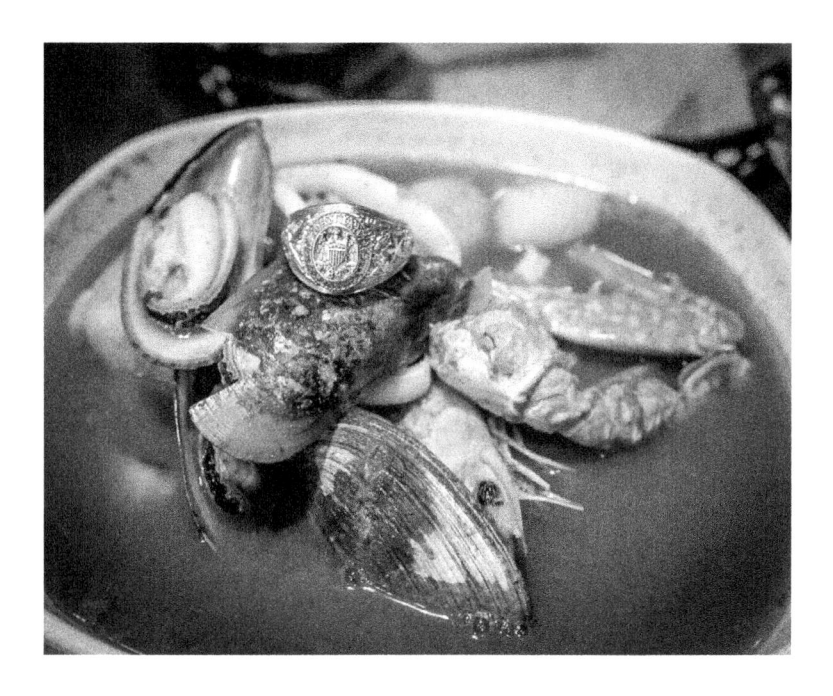

For everyone who is on a high protein diet, seafood is one of the most suggested foods. It has a high-quality protein that is easier to digest for it has less tissue than beef, pork, lamb, or poultry. This is why: cooked fish and seafood are easy to flake without further slicing. Besides that, seafood is also low calorie. There is no reason not to include seafood in the meal plan.

Yield: 4

Preparation Time: 20 minutes

List of Ingredients:

- 1 cup broccoli florets
- ¾ cup chopped mushroom
- ¾ cup fresh shrimps
- ½ cup fish fillet
- 2 tbsp. diced tomatoes
- ½ tsp. olive oil
- ¼ cup diced onion
- ½ cup water
- 1 cup skim milk
- 1 tbsp. coconut flour
- ½ tsp. pepper
- ½ tsp. salt

MMMMMMMMMMMMMMMMMMMMMMMMMMMMMM

Methods:

1. Peel the shrimp, then discard the heads. Set aside.
2. Cut the fish fillet into cubes then set aside.
3. Preheat a skillet over medium heat, then pour olive oil into the skillet.
4. Stir in the chopped onion then sauté until wilted and translucent.
5. Add the fresh shrimp, cubed fish, mushroom, and broccoli to the skillet then pour the water into the skillet. Bring to a boil.
6. Meanwhile, combine the skim milk with coconut flour in a bowl. Stir until incorporated then set aside.
7. When the soup is boiled, season with salt and pepper then pour the skim milk and coconut flour mixture into the skillet. Stir well and bring to a simmer.
8. Once it is done, remove from heat then transfer the soup to a serving bowl.
9. Serve and enjoy immediately.

(27) Spinach Creamy Chicken

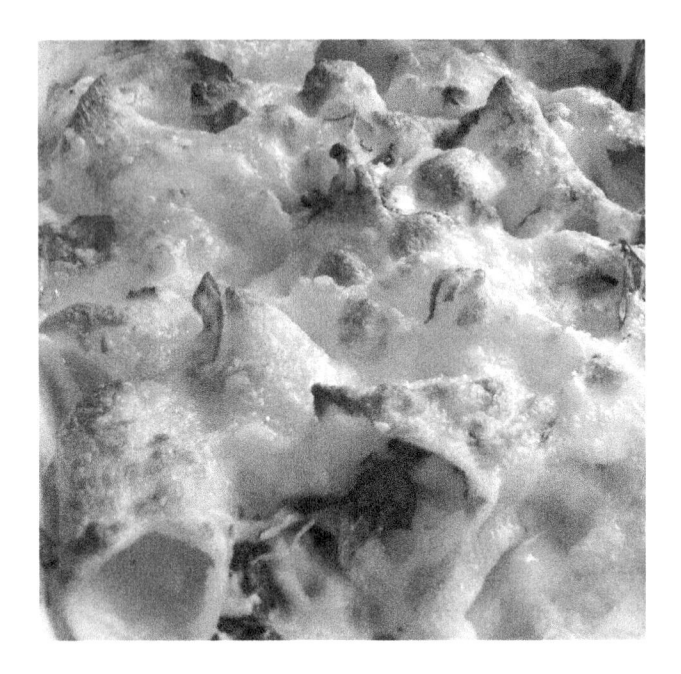

This casserole is so cheesy and creamy. Contained healthy proteins and vitamins that will help you to cultivate a better metabolism, this casserole is a great choice for both lunch and dinner. Another good point of this casserole is that it can be cooked ahead. Cover with aluminum foil and chill in the fridge. Once you want to consume, you just have to microwave it and enjoy it warm. It saves you time and energy.

Yield: 4

Preparation Time: 45 minutes

List of Ingredients:

- 2 cups chopped spinach
- 2 cups ground chicken
- ½ cup non-fat yogurt
- ½ cup skim milk
- 2 organic eggs
- 1 cup grated mozzarella cheese
- 2 tsp. garlic powder

MMMMMMMMMMMMMMMMMMMMMMMMMMMMMM

Methods:

1. Preheat an oven to 350 °F and coat a casserole dish with cooking spray.
2. Preheat a steamer then steam for a few seconds or until the spinach is wilted. Remove from the steamer and set aside.
3. Crack the eggs into a bowl. Whisk well.
4. Season the eggs with garlic powder, then pour skim milk and not-fat yogurt into the bowl. Whisk until incorporated.
5. Arrange the spinach in the bottom of the prepared casserole dish then spread ground chicken over the spinach.
6. Pour the egg mixture over the chicken then sprinkle grated Mozzarella cheese on top.
7. Bake the chicken casserole for approximately 45 minutes or until the egg is set.
8. Once it is done, remove from the oven then let it cool for a few minutes.
9. Serve and enjoy.

(28) Simple Tuna Garlic

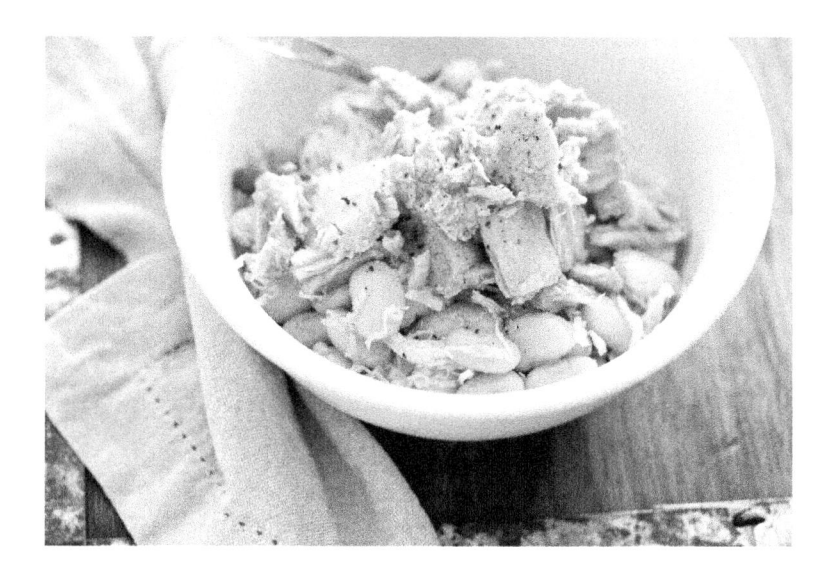

Tuna has a list of nutritional value. However, some people don't like the fishy smell. Adding garlic and other herbs to the dish will disguise the aroma. Moreover, it will also enhance the taste. Serve this tuna with mashed potato or whole-wheat bread and enjoy with any kind of healthy sauce as you desire.

Yield: 4

Preparation Time: 20 minutes

List of Ingredients:

- 2 cups tuna chunks
- 1 tsp. olive oil
- 2 tsp. minced garlic
- 1 cup low sodium chicken broth
- 1 tbsp. Worcestershire sauce
- 1 tbsp. white vinegar
- 1 tsp. mustard
- ½ tsp. pepper
- ¼ cup diced tomatoes

MMMMMMMMMMMMMMMMMMMMMMMMMMMMMMM

Methods:

1. Preheat a skillet over medium heat, then pour olive oil into the skillet.
2. Stir in minced garlic then sauté until lightly golden and aromatic.
3. Add tuna chunks to the skillet, then season with Worcestershire sauce, white vinegar, mustard, and pepper.
4. Pour the chicken broth over the tuna then cook until the liquid is completely absorbed into the tuna.
5. Add the diced tomatoes on top then stir until the tomatoes are wilted.
6. Remove the skillet from heat then serve.
7. Enjoy!

(29) Black Beans Smooth Soup

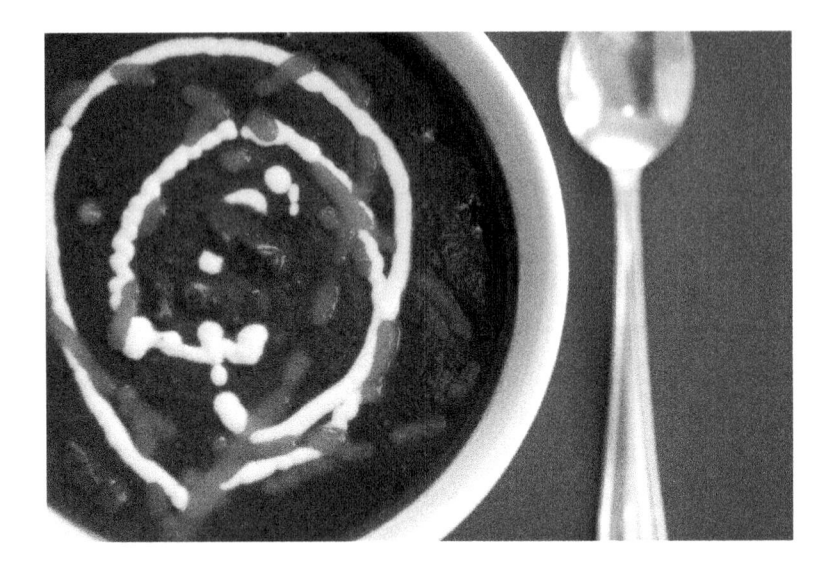

If you are looking for a healthy but tasty soup, for sure, this soup is an excellent option. Beans and chicken, both good sources of protein, are perfect to be included in your meal plan. For a vegetarian option, you can remove the chicken and chicken broth and replace them with vegetables and water. Adding some lemon juice to the soup will also give it a better aroma. Enjoy!

Yield: 4

Preparation Time: 45 minutes

List of Ingredients:

- 1 cup cooked black beans
- 1 cup low-sodium chicken broth
- 1 cup water
- ½ cup diced tomatoes
- ½ tsp. cilantro
- ½ cup coconut milk
- 1 cup ground chicken
- 2 tbsp. chopped onion
- ¼ tsp. pepper
- ¼ tsp. nutmeg

MMMMMMMMMMMMMMMMMMMMMMMMMMMMMM

Methods:

1. Pour water and low-sodium chicken broth into a pot then bring the mixture to a boil.
2. Add black beans and ground chicken, season with cilantro, chopped onion, pepper, and nutmeg. Cook until it becomes thicker.
3. Add diced tomatoes and pour coconut milk into the pot. Bring to a simmer.
4. Remove from heat then let it warm.
5. Using an immersion blender, blend the soup until smooth then transfer to a serving bowl.
6. Serve and enjoy immediately.

Chapter VI: Stage Four-Dinner

MMMMMMMMMMMMMMMMMMMMMMMMMMMMMM

(30) Lentil Loaf Barbecue

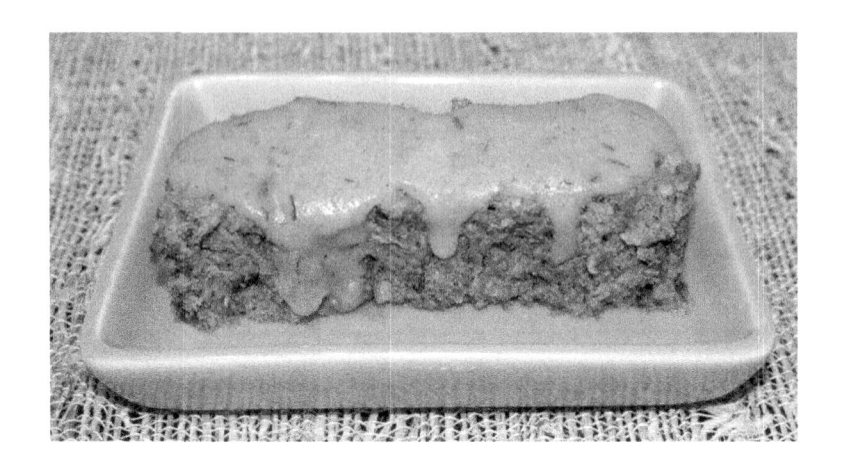

Known as a superfood, lentils contain lots of health benefits for the body. It is rich in protein that is very necessary for everyone who has just had a gastric bypass. Moreover, lentils are good to control diabetes, improve digestion, heart health, and weight management. As a variation, you can shape the loaf into small balls or fritters. Enjoy the healthy lentils with roasted or sautéed vegetables.

Yield: 4

Preparation Time: 60 minutes

List of Ingredients:

- 1 cup cooked lentils
- 1 cup chopped onion
- 2 tsp. minced garlic
- 1 tbsp. whole-wheat flour
- 3 tbsp. flax seeds
- 1 cup tomato paste
- ¼ cup apple cider vinegar
- 2½ tbsp. Worcestershire sauce
- 1 tbsp. hickory smoke
- 1½ tsp. garlic powder
- 1 tsp. onion powder
- 1 cup water

MMMMMMMMMMMMMMMMMMMMMMMMMMMMMM

Methods:

1. Combine the tomato paste with apple cider vinegar, Worcestershire sauce, hickory smoke, garlic powder, onion powder, and water in a saucepan. Stir well.
2. Bring to a simmer until the mixture is completely dissolved. Remove from the heat, then set the sauce aside.
3. Preheat an oven to 350 °F and line a small loaf pan with aluminum foil then set aside.
4. Place the cooked lentils, chopped onion, minced garlic, whole-wheat flour, and flax seeds in a bowl then mix well.
5. Transfer the lentil mixture to the prepared loaf pan then spread evenly.
6. Bake the lentil loaf for approximately 40 minutes or until firm. Insert a skewer into the loaf. If the skewer comes out clean, it means that the loaf has been done.
7. Remove the lentil loaf from the oven then let it cool for a few minutes.
8. Transfer the lentil loaf to a serving dish then drizzle the sauce on top.
9. Serve and enjoy right away.

(31) Sweet Brown Chicken Breast

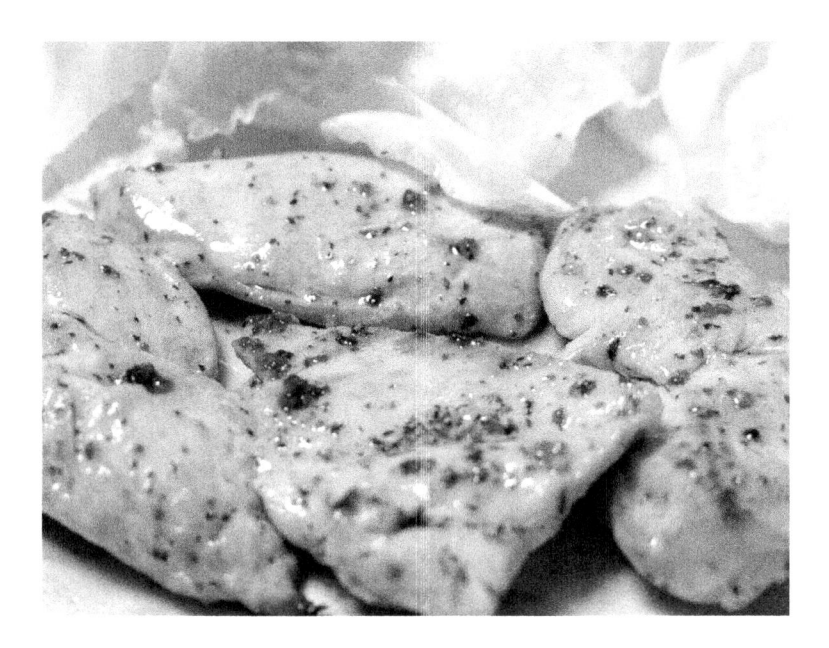

The secret key to the delicacy of this dish is the marinade process. It is true that this chicken bread will taste delicious with a short period of marinade time. However, it, for sure, will be more special if you can marinade it for a longer time. Marinate the chicken for at least 4 hours to overnight will ensure the chicken to be completely seasoned. It will be better if you can add more herbs or seasoning to the rubbing mixture. Good luck.

Yield: 4

Preparation Time: 30 minutes

List of Ingredients:

- 1 lb. boneless chicken breast
- 2 tsp. olive oil
- 3 tsp. garlic powder
- 2 tsp. brown sugar
- ½ tsp. pepper

MMMMMMMMMMMMMMMMMMMMMMMMMMMMMMMM

Methods:

1. Place the garlic powder, pepper, and brown sugar in a bowl, then mix well.
2. Rub the chicken breast with the spice mixture then set aside.
3. Preheat a saucepan over medium heat, then pour olive oil into the saucepan.
4. Once it is hot, add chicken to the saucepan then cook until the chicken is no longer pink and the brown sugar is melted.
5. Transfer the cooked chicken to a serving dish then drizzle the liquid on top.
6. Serve and enjoy.

(32) Sweet Sour Beef Tender with Broccoli

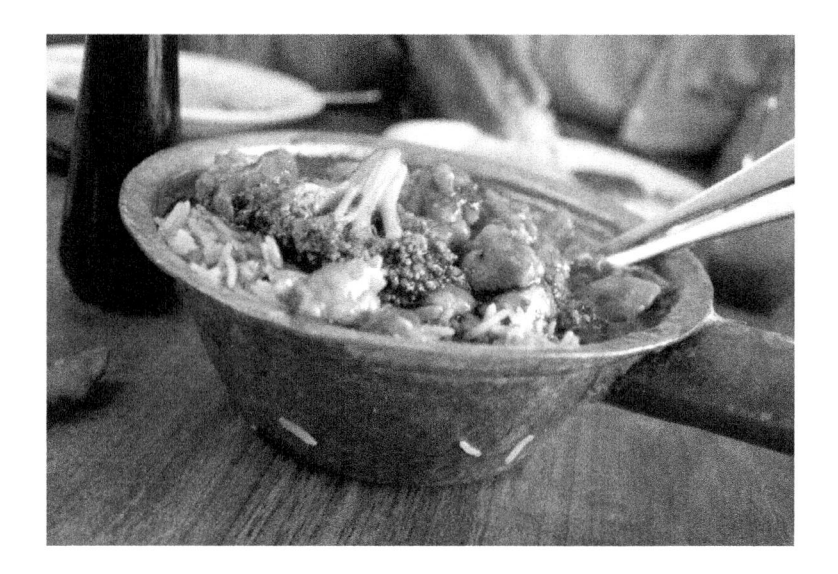

As a great antioxidant, broccoli has become one of the most loved vegetables in the world. Cook the beef until tender, then stir in the broccoli florets at the last step. This will keep the broccoli to be crunchy and tasty. Cut the beef as thin as possible to reduce the cooking time. Besides beef, chicken or pork will work well for this recipe, too!

Yield: 4

Preparation Time: 60 minutes

List of Ingredients:

- ¾ lb. cooked beef tenderloin
- 1 ½ cups broccoli florets
- 1 tsp. olive oil
- ½ cup chopped onion
- ½ tsp. pepper
- ½ tsp. nutmeg
- ¾ cup water
- ¼ cup tomato puree
- 2 tbsp. low-sodium soy sauce

MMMMMMMMMMMMMMMMMMMMMMMMMMMMMMM

Methods:

1. Cut the cooked beef into thin slices, then set aside.
2. Preheat a skillet over medium heat then pour olive oil into the skillet.
3. Stir in the chopped onion then sauté until translucent and aromatic.
4. Add the sliced beef to the skillet then season with pepper and nutmeg.
5. Pour the water into the skillet then drizzle tomato puree and soy sauce over the beef. Bring to a boil.
6. Once it is boiling, add the broccoli florets to the skillet then stir until wilted.
7. Transfer the beef and broccoli to a serving dish then serve.
8. Enjoy!

(33) Turkey Soup Mushroom

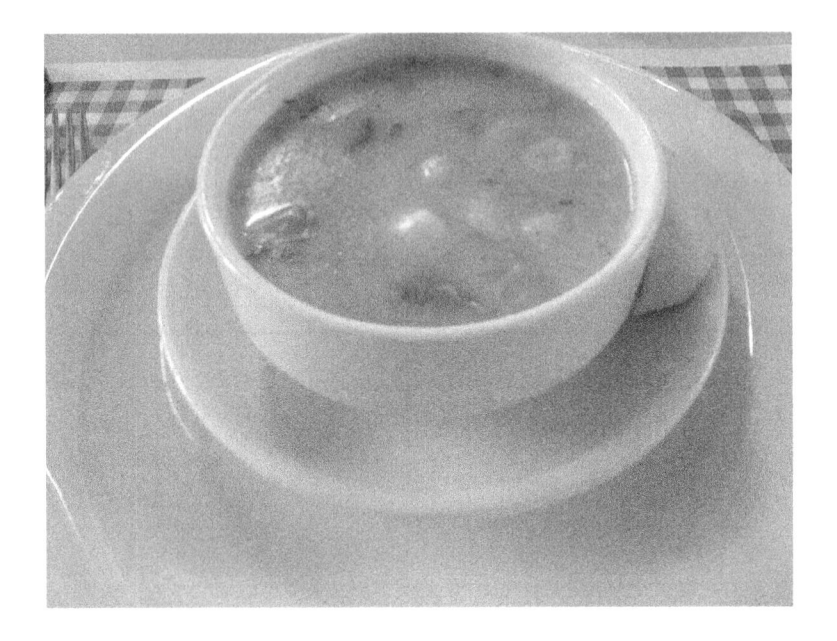

This soup is very light. However, you don't need to worry about the content. The turkey and mushroom provide lots of protein and other essential nutrients. Other than that, the additional ingredients like chicken base, onion, and garlic add a tempting aroma to the dish.

Yield: 1

Preparation Time: 30 minutes

List of Ingredients:

- ½ tsp. olive oil
- 1 tbsp. diced onion
- 2 tbsp. diced mushroom
- 2 tbsp. ground turkey
- 1 tsp. chicken base
- ½ tsp. minced garlic
- ¼ tsp. pepper
- 2 cups water

MMMMMMMMMMMMMMMMMMMMMMMMMMMMMMMM

Methods:

1. Preheat a skillet over medium heat then pour olive oil into it.
2. Stir in the chopped onion and minced garlic, then sauté until wilted and aromatic.
3. Add the diced mushroom and ground turkey, then stir until the turkey is no longer pink.
4. Pour the water into the skillet then add the chicken base and pepper. Stir well.
5. Bring to a boil and once it is boiled, reduce the heat and cook until the gravy has reduced to a half.
6. Transfer to a serving dish then enjoy warm.

(34) Baked Chicken Balls with Cheese Sauce

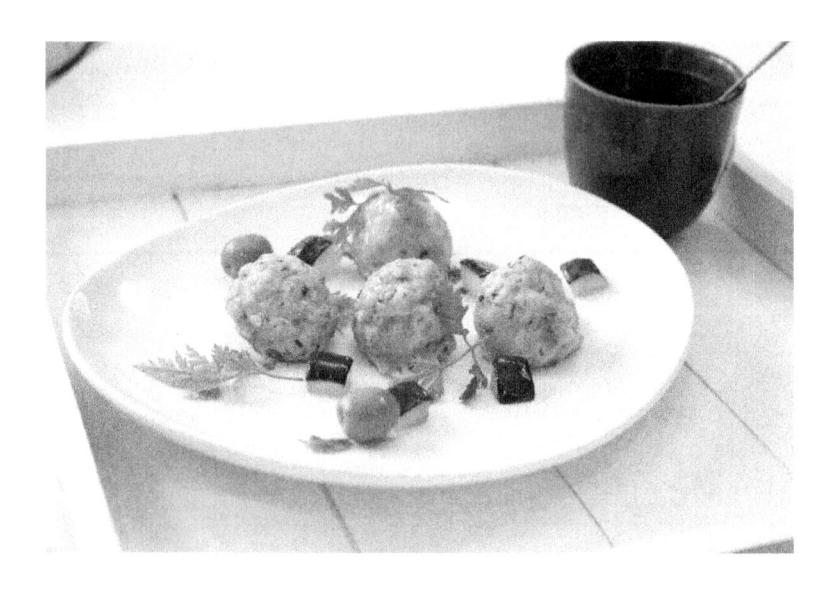

If you want to find an easy but tasty meal recipe, this recipe is exactly a right choice. Cheese, milk, egg, and special spices present a scrumptious dish that will be loved by both kids and adults. Not only for lunch or dinner, but this dish is also great to be enjoyed between the meal times. If you have spare time, you can make the baked chicken balls ahead then chill in the fridge up to 3 days or freeze up to months. However, do not prepare the cheese sauce ahead because it will taste best if it is cooked just before serving.

Yield: 4

Preparation Time: 30 minutes

List of Ingredients:

- 2 lbs. lean ground chicken
- 2 tbsp. coconut flour
- 2 organic eggs
- 1 tbsp. diced celery
- 1 tsp. onion powder
- 1 tsp. garlic powder
- 1 tsp. olive oil
- ¼ cup diced onion
- ½ cup non-fat cheese
- 1 cup skim milk
- 1 tbsp. coconut flour
- ¼ tsp. pepper

MMMMMMMMMMMMMMMMMMMMMMMMMMMMMM

Methods:

1. Place the lean ground chicken, coconut flour, and eggs in a food processor.
2. Season with onion powder and garlic powder then process until smooth.
3. Transfer the smooth mixture to a bowl then add diced celery to the mixture. Mix until combined.
4. Preheat an oven to 350 °F and line a baking sheet with parchment paper.
5. Shape the chicken mixture into balls forms then arrange on the prepared baking sheet.
6. Bake the chicken balls for approximately 20 minutes. Stir once every 5 minutes.
7. Meanwhile, preheat a skillet over medium heat then pour olive oil into the skillet.
8. Stir in diced onion then sauté until translucent and aromatic.
9. Pour skim milk into the skillet then season with pepper.
10. Cut the non-fat cheese into cubes then add to the mixture. Cook until the cheese is melted.
11. Add coconut flour to the skillet then bring to a simmer. Remove from heat.

12. Once the chicken balls are done, remove from the oven then transfer the baked chicken balls to a serving dish.
13. Drizzle cheese sauce over the chicken balls then serve.
14. Enjoy right away.

(35) Sautéed Shrimps Garlic

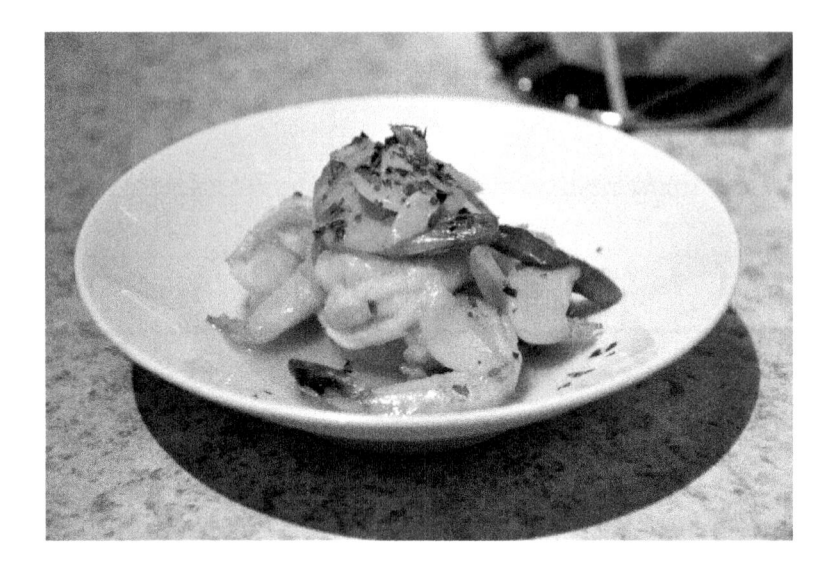

Shrimp is a kind of seafood that is rich in protein, but low in carbohydrates and fats. The shrimp has a natural sweetness that will make the food you cook with tastes wonderful. The key to a firm and crunchy cooked shrimps texture is the cooking time. Shrimp does not need a long period of time to be cooked. Add the shrimp at the last minute and cook just until pink. Besides shrimp, this recipe will also work well for squid, clam, and crab.

Yield: 4

Preparation Time: 30 minutes

List of Ingredients:

- ½ tsp. olive oil
- 1 lb. fresh shrimps
- 2 tsp. minced garlic
- 1 tsp. fish sauce
- ¼ cup diced tomatoes

MMMMMMMMMMMMMMMMMMMMMMMMMMMMMMM

Methods:

1. Peel the shrimp then discard the heads. Set aside.
2. Preheat a skillet over medium heat, then pour olive oil into it.
3. Once the oil is hot, stir in minced garlic, then sauté until wilted and aromatic.
4. Add the peeled shrimp to the skillet, then season with fish sauce. Mix well.
5. Stir in the diced tomatoes and cook until just wilted.
6. Transfer the sautéed shrimp to a serving dish then serve.
7. Enjoy!

(36) Beans Soup with Enchilada Sauce

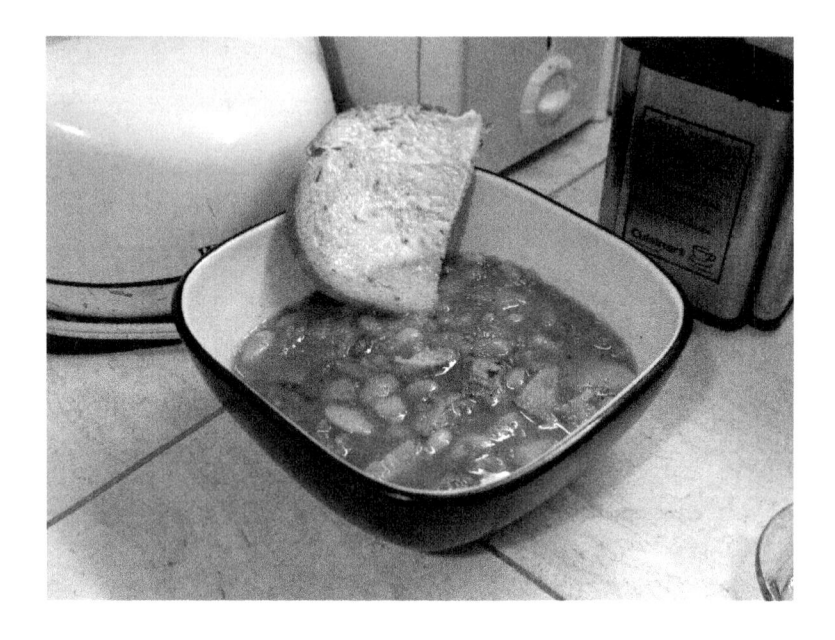

Beans are not only nutritious but also delicious. This recipe uses pinto beans as the main ingredient. However, you can change them out with any kinds of beans that are available in your lovely kitchen. Kidney beans, black beans, or white beans are a great substitute. Cooking this recipe with varying kinds of beans quite often is really suggested. Don't worry; all the beans are a good source of fiber and protein. Besides, the beans are also cholesterol-free, fat-free, and sodium-free.

Yield: 4

Preparation Time: 60 minutes

List of Ingredients:

- 1 cup pinto beans, soaked overnight
- ½ cup tomato puree
- 1½ cups Enchilada red sauce
- 3 cups water
- ¾ tsp. cumin
- ¼ tsp. salt
- ¼ tsp. black pepper
- ½ tsp. olive oil
- 2 tbsp. chopped onion

MMMMMMMMMMMMMMMMMMMMMMMMMMMMMMM

Methods:

1. Place the beans and water in a pot then bring everything to a boil.
2. Once it is boiling, reduce the heat then cook the pinto beans until tender. Usually, the water will be reduced by more than half.
3. When the beans are tender, remove them from the heat then set aside.
4. Preheat a skillet over medium heat then pour olive oil into it.
5. Once it is hot, stir in chopped onion then sauté until wilted and aromatic.
6. Pour the cooked beans together with the liquid into the skillet, then add the tomato sauce and Enchilada red sauce to the skillet.
7. Season with cumin, salt, and black pepper then bring to boil.
8. Once it is boiling, reduce the heat then cook for another 3 minutes or until the gravy is thick.
9. Transfer the cooked beans together with the gravy to a serving bowl then serve.
10. Enjoy warm.

(37) Tomato Beef Casserole

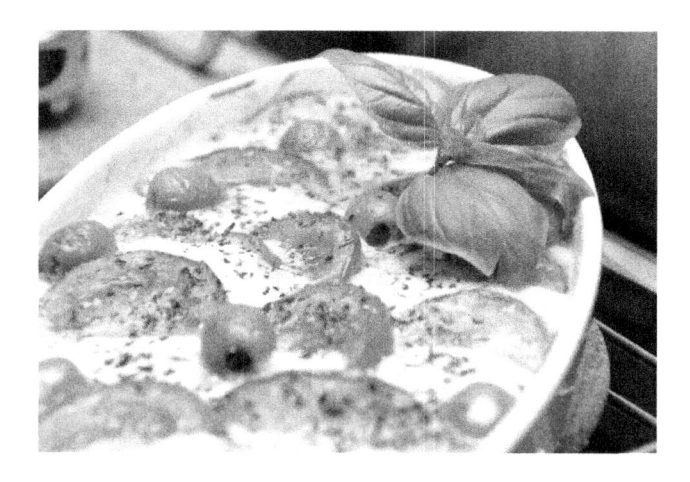

This casserole is really a great choice. Beef, tomato, cucumber, and cheese are super ingredients that will generate an awesome dish. In less than an hour, you can serve a tasty and healthy casserole for your beloved family. Adding some other ingredients, such as mushroom, spinach, cauliflower, and much more, will enhance the taste and the nutrient content. Not to mention, help create a better appearance. For later usage, wait until the casserole is cool then cover with aluminum foil. Chill in the fridge up to 4 days and microwave whenever you want to enjoy it.

Yield: 4

Preparation Time: 45 minutes

List of Ingredients:

- 2 cups lean ground beef
- ½ tsp. olive oil
- 1½ cup diced tomatoes
- ½ cup cubed cucumber
- 1 cup grated Mozzarella cheese
- 3 organic eggs
- ½ cup skim milk
- ½ tsp. pepper
- 2 tsp. garlic powder

MMMMMMMMMMMMMMMMMMMMMMMMMMMMMMM

Methods:

1. Preheat an oven to 350 °F and coat a casserole dish with cooking spray.
2. Crack the eggs into a bowl.
3. Add the pepper and garlic powder to the bowl, then pour in some skim milk.
4. Preheat a skillet over medium heat, then pour olive oil into the skillet.
5. Once it is hot, stir in lean ground beef then sauté until brown.
6. Remove the beef from heat then pour the egg mixture over the beef. Stir until combined.
7. Transfer the beef and the liquid to the prepared casserole dish then sprinkle cucumber and tomatoes over the beef.
8. Top with grated Mozzarella cheese then bake for approximately 45-55 minutes or until the liquid is set.
9. Once it is done, take the casserole dish out of the oven then let it sit.
10. Serve and enjoy right away.

(38) Savory Steamed Fish

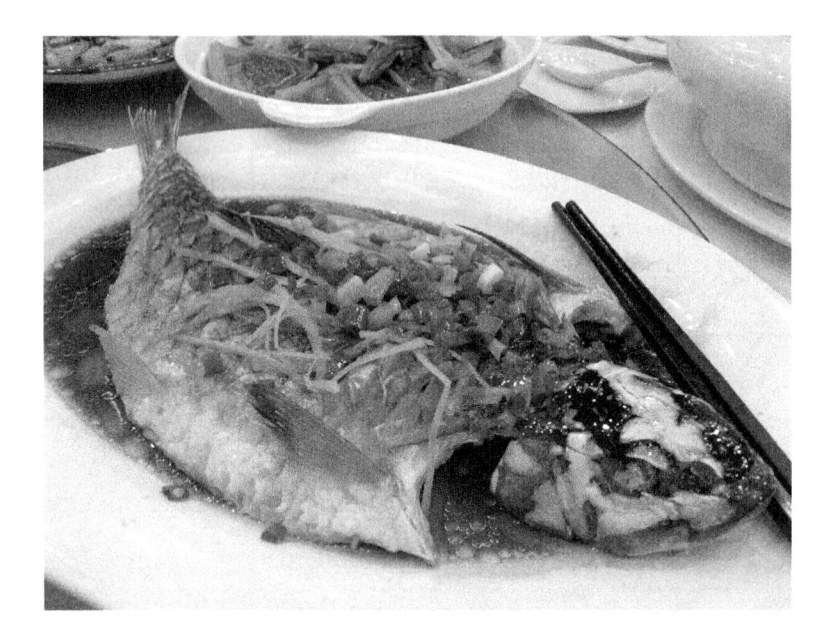

Fish is already savory. With some additional herbs, the delicacy of fish can reach its maximum. This steamed fish uses traditional herbs that will not only enhance the taste of the fish but also serve a tempting aroma. Without involving oil in this recipe, this dish is considered as a low-fat meal. Enjoy this dish for lunch or dinner with a cup of brown rice. If you like a spicy taste, add some green or red chili flakes to this dish.

Yield: 4

Preparation Time: 15 minutes

List of Ingredients:

- 2 lbs. fresh fish
- 3 tsp. minced garlic
- 1 tsp. cumin
- 2 tbsp. lemon juice
- 2 lemongrasses
- ¼ cup fresh basil
- 2 tbsp. chopped leek

MMMMMMMMMMMMMMMMMMMMMMMMMMMMMMMMM

Methods:

1. Preheat a steamer over medium heat and prepare a baking dish.
2. Place the minced garlic, cumin, lemon grasses, and basil in a food processor.
3. Add the lemon juice to the food processor then process until smooth.
4. Rub the fish with the spice mixture then place in the prepared baking dish.
5. Place the baking dish in the steamer then steam the fish for 15 minutes or until the fish is easy to flake.
6. Once it is done, remove the baking dish from the steamer and let it sit.
7. Transfer the steamed fish together with the liquid to a serving dish.
8. Sprinkle chopped leek over the fish then serve.
9. Enjoy!

(39) Mixed Vegetables Tender

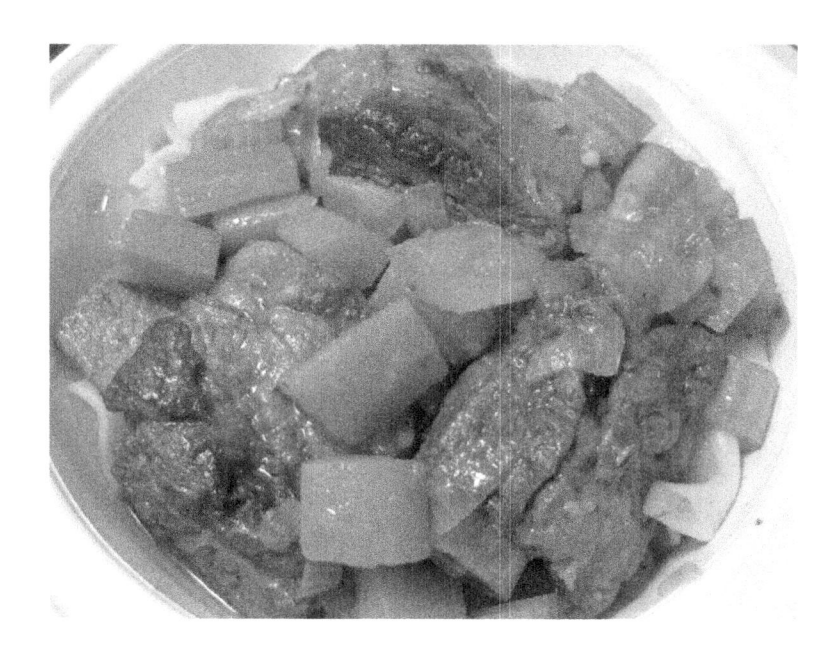

There is no doubt that vegetables contain great nutrients for the body. However, some people think that vegetables do not taste good. This recipe, for sure, breaks the opinion. These mixed vegetables generate a delicious dish that you never imagine before. The fish sauce in this dish gives a great savory taste while the soy sauce provides a better color. Do not overcook the vegetables to keep the crunchy texture and the natural sweetness.

Yield: 4

Preparation Time: 15 minutes

List of Ingredients:

- ¼ cup sliced carrots
- ¼ cup baby corn
- 1 cup chopped green collard
- ½ cup cauliflower florets
- 2 tbsp. chopped leek
- 1 tsp. olive oil
- 2 tsp. minced garlic
- ¼ tsp. pepper
- 1 tbsp. fish sauce
- 1 tbsp. low-sodium soy sauce
- 2 tbsp. tomato puree
- ½ cup water

MMMMMMMMMMMMMMMMMMMMMMMMMMMMMM

Methods:

1. Preheat a skillet over medium heat then pour olive oil into the skillet.
2. Once it is hot, stir in minced garlic then sauté until aromatic and lightly golden.
3. Next, add the sliced carrots and baby corn then sauté until wilted.
4. Pour water into the skillet then season the vegetables with pepper, fish sauce, soy sauce, and tomato puree. Mix well and bring to boil.
5. Once it is boiled, stir in the green collard and cauliflower florets then cook until the vegetables are wilted. Stir well.
6. Once it is done, transfer the cooked mixed vegetables to a serving dish, then enjoy right away.

Chapter VII: Stage Four-Snack and Dessert

MMMMMMMMMMMMMMMMMMMMMMMMMMMMMM

(40) Mango Tropical Salsa

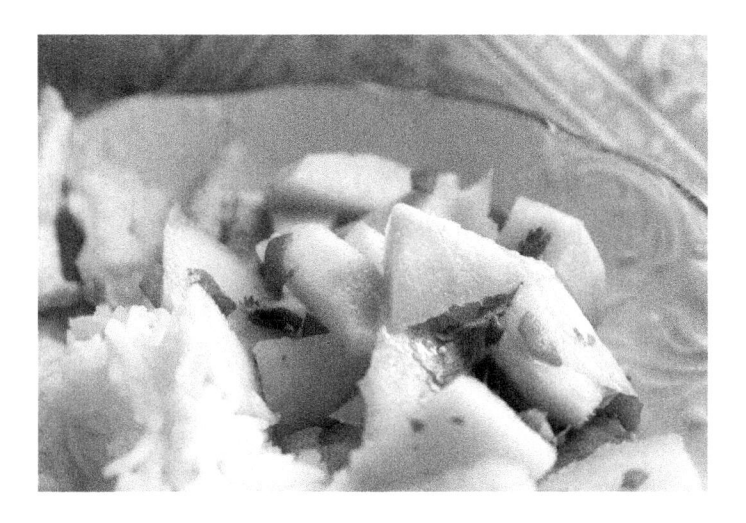

It is recommended to enjoy this snack with tortilla chips or as a condiment on baked chicken, beef, pork, and fish. Always choose the ripe mangoes that are fresh and still have a firm texture. The ripe, but not very soft mangoes will be easier to peel and cut than the mushy ones. For some variations, you can add or substitute the fruits with the other fruits, as you desired. Pineapples, apples, or avocados are also good great fruits for this recipe.

Yield: 4

Preparation Time: 15 minutes

List of Ingredients:

- 2 ripe mangoes
- ½ cup chopped onion
- 2 tbsp. cilantro
- 3 tbsp. lemon juice
- ¼ cup diced tomatoes
- A pinch of salt
- A pinch of pepper

MMMMMMMMMMMMMMMMMMMMMMMMMMMMMMM

Methods:

1. Peel the mangoes then cut into small cubes.
2. Place the cubed mangoes in a salad bowl then add chopped onion, cilantro, and diced tomatoes.
3. Sprinkle salt and pepper over the ingredients then drizzle lemon juice on top. Toss to combine.
4. Cover the bowl with the lid then chill the mango mixture in the fridge.
5. Serve and enjoy cold.

(41) Dense Oatmeal Cake

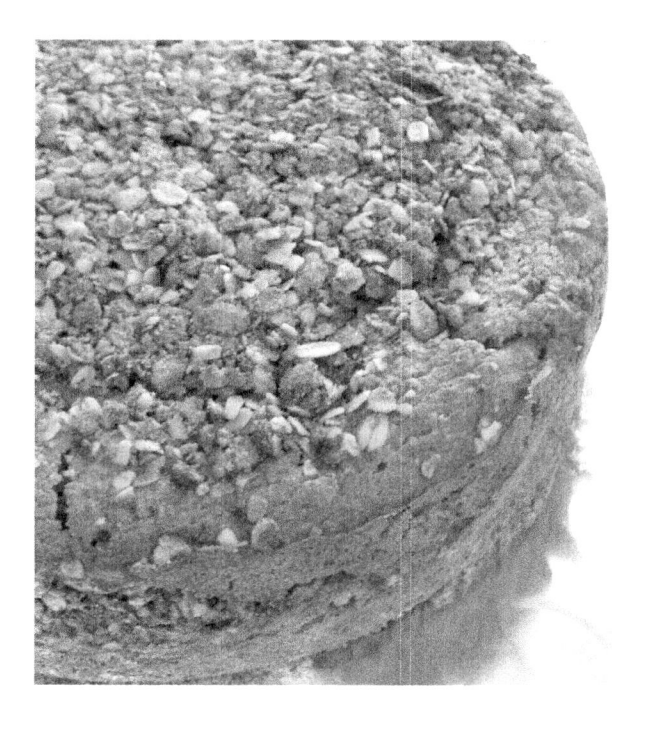

This cake has a dense texture. However, this cake is good as it serves you a good amount of fiber. The brown sugar and cinnamon also provide great flavor and aroma. This cake is best to be served as a nutritious breakfast, re-energizing snack, or tasteful dessert. Chill the cake in the fridge and serve it cold if you want to try something different. For later usage, wrap the cake with aluminum foil and put it in the freezer for months.

Yield: 4

Preparation Time: 40 minutes

List of Ingredients:

- 1 cup rolled oats
- ¾ tsp. baking powder
- ½ cup low-fat buttermilk
- 2 organic eggs
- 4 tbsp. applesauce
- 2 tsp. brown sugar
- 1 tsp. cinnamon

MMMMMMMMMMMMMMMMMMMMMMMMMMMMM

Methods:

1. Preheat an oven to 325 °F and line a small baking pan with parchment paper. Set aside.
2. Combine the rolled oats with baking powder, brown sugar, and cinnamon. Stir well.
3. In another bowl, crack the eggs and add the applesauce and buttermilk. Whisk until incorporated.
4. Pour the liquid mixture over the dry mixture, then whisk until combined.
5. Transfer the mixture to the prepared baking pan. Spread evenly.
6. Bake the cake for approximately 40 minutes or until a skewer that is inserted into the cake comes out clean.
7. Remove from the oven then let the cake cool for a few minutes.
8. Take the cake out from the pan then cut into slices.
9. Serve and enjoy.

(42) Roasted Chickpeas

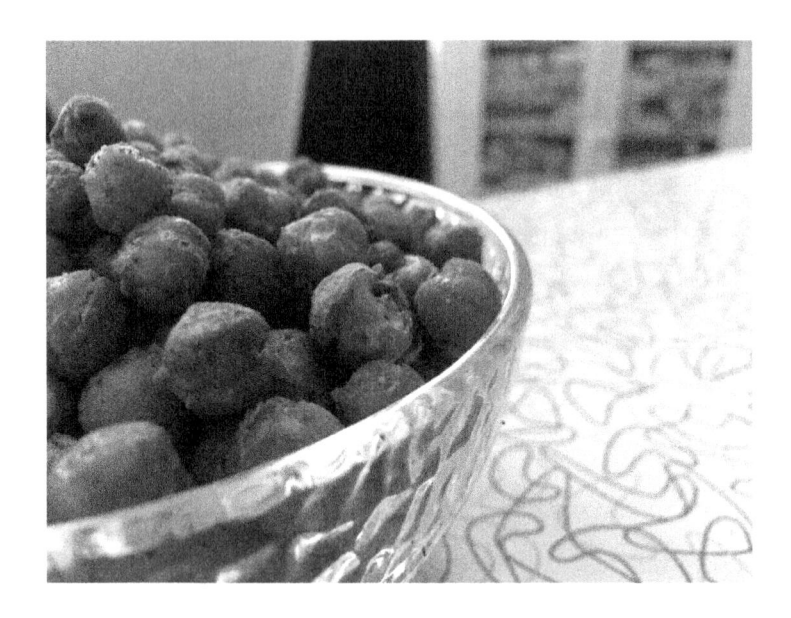

There is no doubt that chickpeas are a superfood. Famous as beneficial legumes, chickpeas are a rich in protein, vitamin, dietary fiber, and mineral. That is why chickpeas have become a favorite among those who want to live healthier. This recipe uses garlic as the main seasoning. However, feel free to enhance the taste of the roasted chickpeas by involving some other seasonings.

Yield: 4

Preparation Time: 45 minutes

List of Ingredients:

- 1 cup chickpeas
- 1 tsp. olive oil
- ½ tsp. garlic powder
- ¼ tsp. cumin
- ½ tsp. salt

MMMMMMMMMMMMMMMMMMMMMMMMMMMMMMM

Methods:

1. Preheat an oven to 350°F and line a baking sheet with parchment paper.
2. Place the chickpeas in a bowl then drizzle olive oil over the chickpeas.
3. Season with garlic powder, cumin, and salt. Toss to combine.
4. Spread the seasoned chickpeas on the prepared baking sheet then roast on the top rack of the oven for approximately 40 minutes.
5. Once it is done, remove from the oven then transfer to a serving dish.
6. Serve and enjoy!

(43) Vanilla Melon Pudding

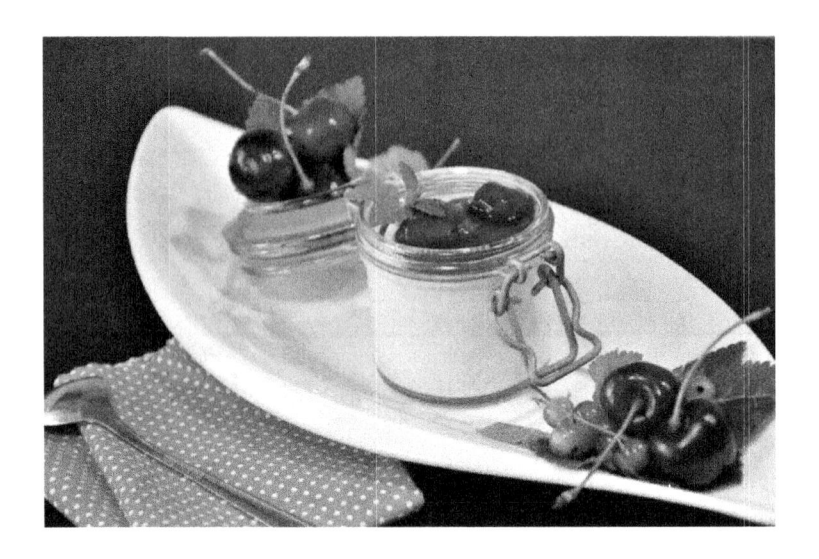

If you are looking for a silky pudding with enough protein content, this recipe is the answer. Made from protein powder, milk, and fresh fruits, there is no doubt that this pudding is not only fresh but also soft, delicious, and nutritious. Do not stick with the fruits in this recipe. Any kind of fruit works well with this recipe. As long as they are fresh, the pudding will taste great.

Yield: 4

Preparation Time: 15 minutes

List of Ingredients:

- 1 ½ cups melon puree
- 2 packages sugar-free Jell-O
- ¼ cup protein powder
- 2 cups skim milk
- ½ cup fresh raspberries

MMMMMMMMMMMMMMMMMMMMMMMMMMMMMMM

Methods:

1. Combine the sugar-free Jell-O with skim milk then pour into a pot.
2. Bring to boil and stir until the Jell-O is completely dissolved.
3. Once the milk and jell-O mixture is boiling, add the protein powder and melon puree. Mix well. Remove from heat.
4. Pour the mixture into 8 small pudding cups then garnish each pudding with fresh raspberries.
5. Chill the puddings in the refrigerator then let them set.
6. Serve and enjoy cold.

(44) Silky Cheese with Cinnamon

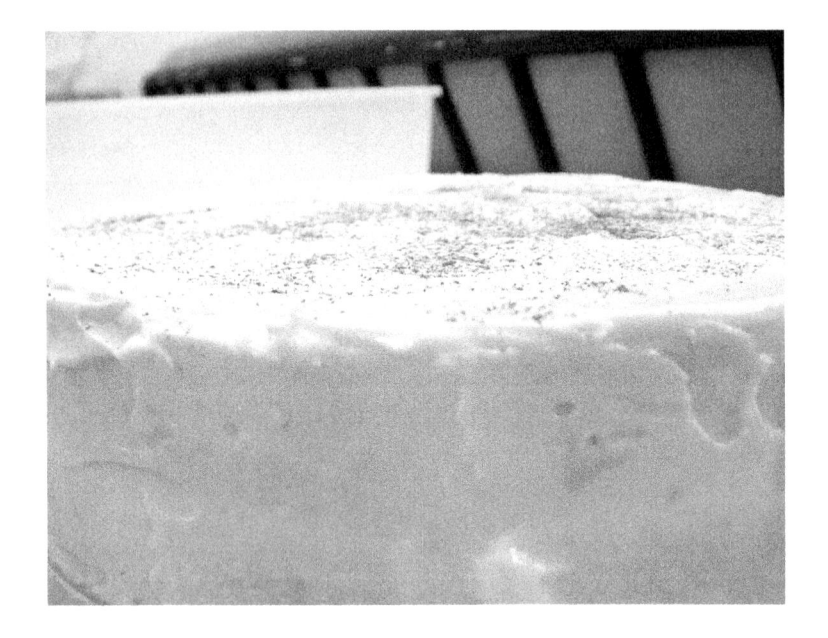

For those who love cheese, this snack will surely make their tongues dance. It is a super creamy and smooth dish that will be a great snack or dessert. The cinnamon does not only give a lovely flavor but also a tempting aroma. Let them stay in the fridge and remove it just before serving. Enjoy cold!

Yield: 4

Preparation Time: 30 minutes

List of Ingredients:

- ¾ cup water
- 1 package sugar-free Jell-O
- ¾ cup non-fat yogurt
- 1 cup non-fat cream cheese
- 1 tbsp. cinnamon

MMMMMMMMMMMMMMMMMMMMMMMMMMMMMM

Methods:

1. Pour the water into a pot, then add sugar-free Jell-O to the pot.
2. Bring to a boil and vigorously stir until the gelatin is completely dissolved in the water.
3. Once it is boiled, remove from the heat and let it warm for a few minutes.
4. Meanwhile, place non-fat cream cheese in a mixing bowl. Using an electric mixer, whisk until softened.
5. Add non-fat yogurt to the mixing bowl then whisk until fluffy and smooth.
6. When the gelatin mixture is warm, slowly pour into the cream cheese and yogurt mixture. Whisk until smooth and incorporated. This may take time.
7. Pour the mixture into 4 pudding cups or 8 small pudding cups then sprinkle cinnamon on top.
8. Let them cool then chill in the fridge until set.
9. Serve and enjoy.

(45) Roasted Cauliflower Garlic

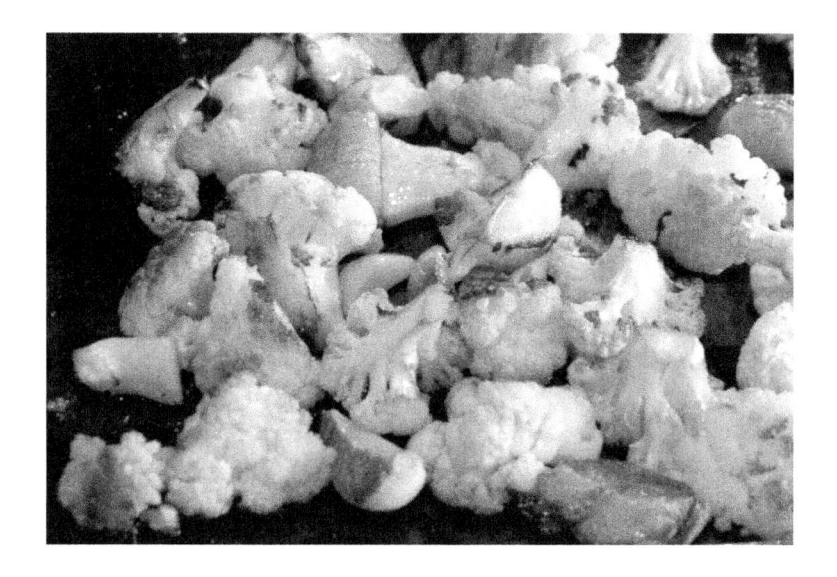

If I have to describe this dish, then I will choose two words. They are simple and healthy. As a good supplier of fiber, vitamins, and mineral, this roasted cauliflower is the best choice to be eaten between the meal times. This roasted cauliflower is already delicious to be enjoyed just the way it is. However, additional tomato sauce, healthy cheese dressing, or homemade barbecue will enhance the taste.

Yield: 4

Preparation Time: 20 minutes

List of Ingredients:

- 2 cups cauliflower florets
- 3 tbsp. avocado oil
- ½ tsp. salt
- ½ tsp. pepper
- 2 tsp. garlic powder

MMMMMMMMMMMMMMMMMMMMMMMMMMMMMMMM

Methods:

1. Preheat an oven to 425 °F and line a baking sheet with parchment paper. Set aside.
2. Place the cauliflower florets in a bowl then drizzle avocado oil over them.
3. Sprinkle the pepper, salt, and garlic then toss to combine.
4. Spread the cauliflower florets on the prepared baking sheet then roast for approximately 15-20 minutes or until the cauliflower florets are tender.
5. Once it is done, remove from the oven then transfer to a serving dish.
6. Serve and enjoy.

(46) Orange Mango Popsicles

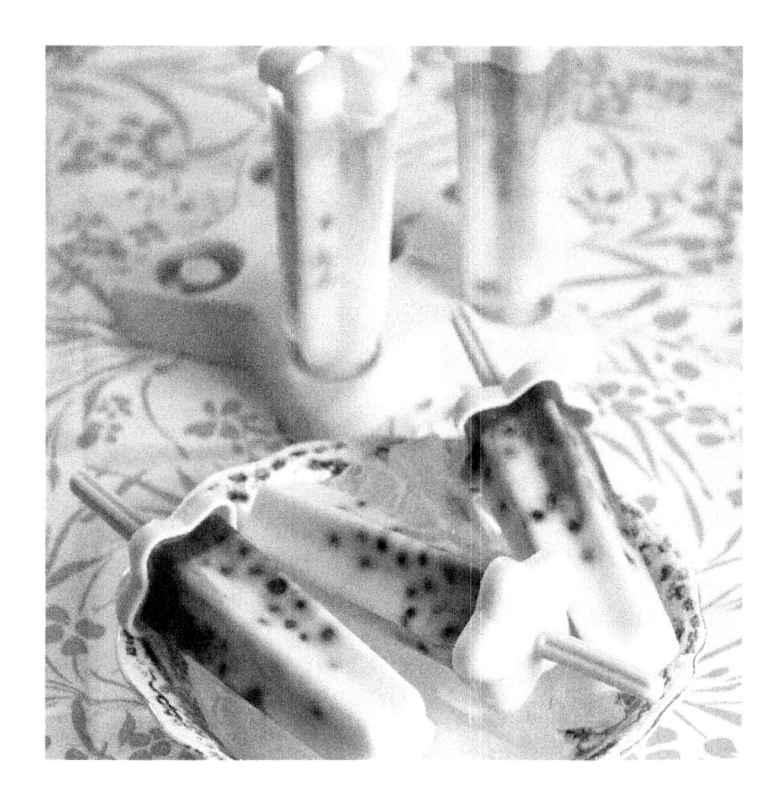

This is another way to enjoy fresh fruits. If you have lots of stock of fruits but have not enough space to store them, making them into popsicles is a brilliant idea. It does not only offer you the same natural sweetness and refreshing sensation with the fresh fruits but also avoid them being overripe. Use your creativity to mix and match ingredients according to the fruits that are available or easy to grab at the moment.

Yield: 4

Preparation Time: 10 minutes

List of Ingredients:

- 2 ripe bananas
- 2 ripe mangoes
- 1 ½ cups unsweetened orange juice

Methods:

1. Peel the bananas then cut into slices. Place in a blender.
2. Peel the mangoes then cut into cubes then also place in the blender.
3. Pour the orange juice over the fruits then blend until incorporated.
4. Pour the mixture into 4 popsicle molds then freeze.
5. Enjoy cold.

(47) Strawberry Sorbet with Ricotta Cheese

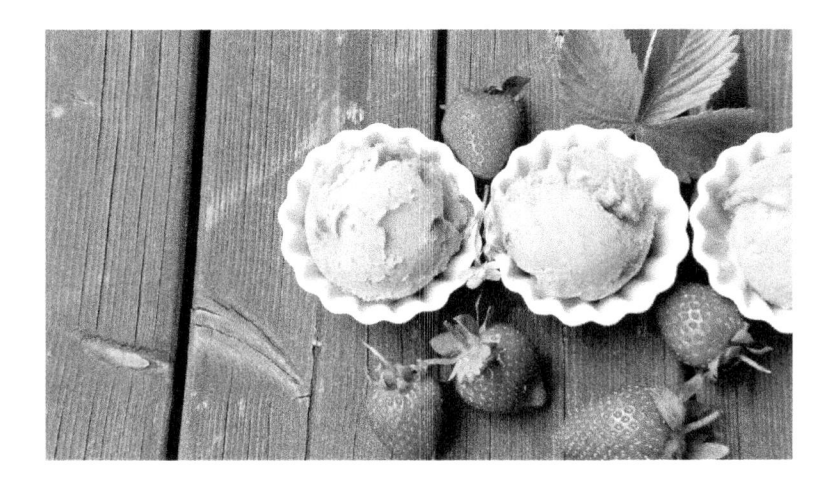

This sorbet only needs three ingredients that are easy to grab. Even, they are usually ready in your refrigerator. The freshness of the fruits is the key to generate a refreshing and fruity taste for this sorbet. Also, fresh fruits will give better color to the sorbet. If strawberry is not in season, you can substitute with pineapple, watermelon, or melon.

Yield: 4

Preparation Time: 21 minutes

List of Ingredients:

- 3 cups frozen strawberries
- ¾ cup skim ricotta
- 1 tbsp. lemon juice

Methods:

1. Place the frozen strawberries in a food processor, then add skim ricotta to the food processor.
2. Drizzle lemon juice over the strawberries then process until smooth.
3. Transfer the strawberry mixture to a container and spread evenly.
4. Store the strawberry sorbet in the freezer and scoop out when you want to consume.
5. Enjoy cold!

(48) Meat Cups and Creamy Topping

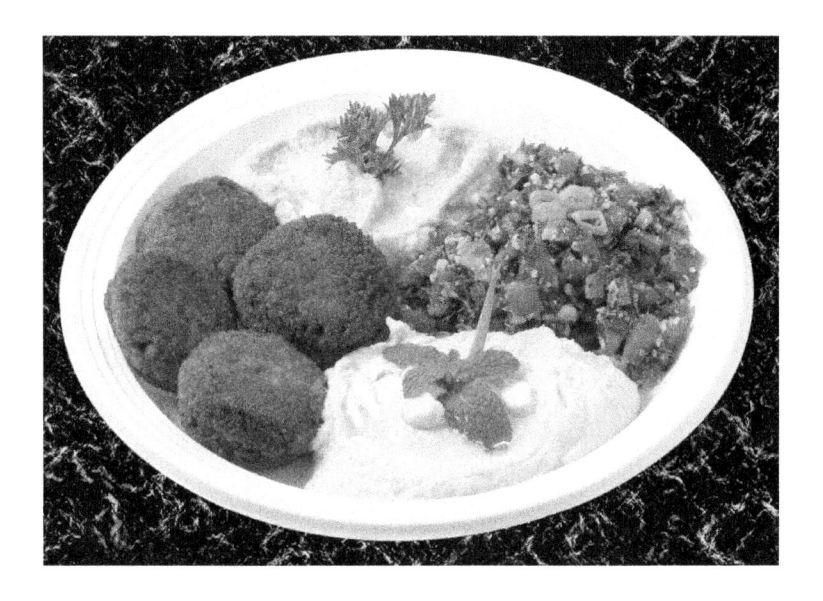

This dish is really fit for everyone who has had a Gastric Bypass surgery. Surely, the smooth texture of turkey and potatoes is good for the new gastric. If you don't like turkey, you can use chicken for this recipe. Of course, organic meat is always the best option. Also, additional vegetables will enrich the health content of this dish. Always grate or puree the vegetables so that they will blend with the ground meat and the mashed potato.

Yield: 4

Preparation Time: 45 minutes

List of Ingredients:

- 1 lb. ground turkey
- ¾ cup grated zucchini
- 2 tbsp. chopped onion
- ½ cup whole-wheat crumbs
- 3 tbsp. ketchup
- ½ lb. potatoes
- 2 tsp. minced garlic
- 1 ½ tbsp. non-fat sour cream
- 1 ½ tbsp. low sodium chicken broth
- 2 tbsp. skim milk
- ½ tsp. pepper
- 1 ½ tbsp. thyme

MMMMMMMMMMMMMMMMMMMMMMMMMMMMMM

Methods:

1. Peel and cut the potatoes, then place them in a steamer.
2. Steam the potatoes for approximately 15 minutes or until the potatoes are tender.
3. Meanwhile, preheat an oven to 350 °F and coat 8 small muffin cups with cooking spray. Set aside.

4. Place the ground turkey in a food processor then add grated zucchini, chopped onion, whole-wheat crumbs, and ketchup to the food processor. Process until smooth.
5. Fill the prepared muffin cups with the turkey mixture then arrange on a baking sheet.
6. Bake the turkey cups for approximately 20 minutes or until the meat cups are cooked through.
7. Remove the turkey cups from the oven then let them cool for a few minutes.
8. While waiting for the turkey cups, take the potatoes from the steamer then place in a bowl.
9. Using a potato masher, mash the potatoes until smooth.
10. Add the minced garlic and non-fat sour cream then pour skim milk and low-sodium chicken broth over the mashed potatoes.
11. Season with pepper and thyme then mix until combined.
12. Take the turkey cups out from the cups then arrange on a serving dish.
13. Top each turkey cups with mashed potatoes then serve.
14. Enjoy!

(49) Lemon Mug Cake

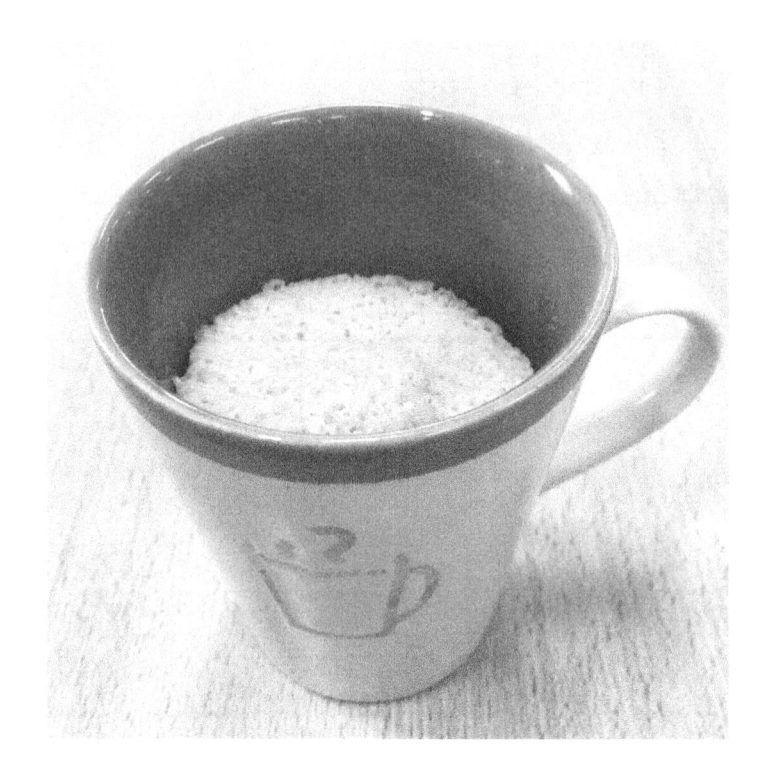

Are you hungry on a hectic workday? Or do you need nutritious breakfast in the busy morning? Then you have to try this mug cake. In only a few minutes, you will get a delicious and aromatic cake to be enjoyed. To enhance the taste, you can involve cheese in this recipe. You have to make sure that you use the non-fat cheese.

Yield: 1

Preparation Time: 5 minutes

List of Ingredients:

- 1 organic egg
- ¼ cup skim milk
- 2 tbsp. applesauce
- 1½ tbsp. avocado oil
- ½ tsp. grated lemon zest
- ½ tbsp. lemon juice
- 2 tbsp. whole grains flour
- 1 scoop protein powder

MMMMMMMMMMMMMMMMMMMMMMMMMMMMMM

Methods:

1. Crack the eggs then place in a measuring cup.
2. Pour skim milk, applesauce, lemon juice, and avocado oil into the cup then mix until incorporated.
3. In a microwave-safe mug, put protein powder, flour, and grated lemon zest then mix well.
4. Pour the liquid mixture into the dry mixture then stir until smooth and incorporated.
5. Place the mug in the microwave then microwave for 2 minutes.
6. Check the doneness of the cake by inserting a skewer into the cake. When it comes out clean, it means that the cake is completely cooked.
7. Microwave for another 30 seconds if it is necessary.
8. Remove the mug cake out from the microwave then let it cool.
9. Serve and enjoy.

About the Author

A native of Indianapolis, Indiana, Valeria Ray found her passion for cooking while she was studying English Literature at Oakland City University. She decided to try a cooking course with her friends and the experience changed her forever. She enrolled at the Art Institute of Indiana which offered extensive courses in the culinary Arts. Once Ray dipped her toe in the cooking world, she never looked back.

When Valeria graduated, she worked in French restaurants in the Indianapolis area until she became the head chef at one of the 5-star establishments in the area. Valeria's attention to taste and visual detail caught the eye of a local business person who expressed an interest in publishing her recipes. Valeria began her secondary career authoring cookbooks and e-books which she tackled with as much talent and gusto as her first career. Her passion for food leaps off the page of her books which have colourful anecdotes and stunning pictures of dishes she has prepared herself.

Valeria Ray lives in Indianapolis with her husband of 15 years, Tom, her daughter, Isobel and their loveable Golden Retriever, Goldy. Valeria enjoys cooking special dishes in her large, comfortable kitchen where the family gets involved in preparing meals. This successful, dynamic chef is an inspiration to culinary students and novice cooks everywhere.

Author's Afterthoughts

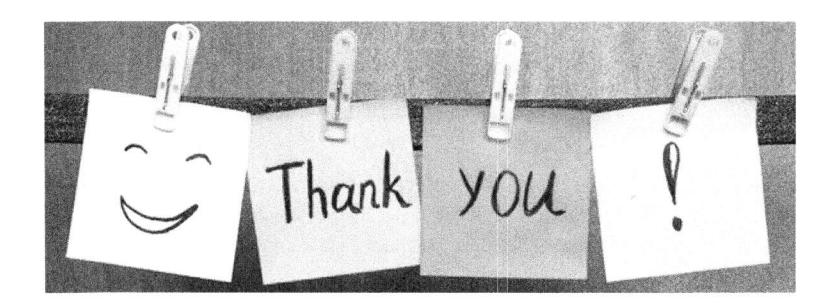

Thank you for Purchasing my book and taking the time to read it from front to back. I am always grateful when a reader chooses my work and I hope you enjoyed it!

With the vast selection available online, I am touched that you chose to be purchasing my work and take valuable time out of your life to read it. My hope is that you feel you made the right decision.

I very much would like to know what you thought of the book. Please take the time to write an honest and informative review on Amazon.com. Your experience and opinions will be of great benefit to me and those readers looking to make an informed choice.

With much thanks,

Valeria Ray

Printed in Great Britain
by Amazon